Building Your Academic Research Digital Identity

Margaret Rush Dreker • Kyle James Downey
Editors

Building Your Academic Research Digital Identity

A Step-Wise Guide to Cultivating Your Academic Research Career Online

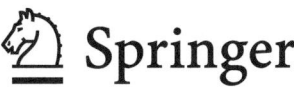
Springer

Editors
Margaret Rush Dreker
Medical Librarian
Hackensack Meridian School of Medicine
Nutley, NJ, USA

Kyle James Downey
College of Nursing & School of Health and Medical Sciences Librarian
Seton Hall University
Montclair, NJ, USA

ISBN 978-3-031-50316-0   ISBN 978-3-031-50317-7 (eBook)
https://doi.org/10.1007/978-3-031-50317-7

© The Editor(s) (if applicable) and The Author(s), under exclusive license to Springer Nature Switzerland AG 2023, corrected publication 2024
This work is subject to copyright. All rights are solely and exclusively licensed by the Publisher, whether the whole or part of the material is concerned, specifically the rights of translation, reprinting, reuse of illustrations, recitation, broadcasting, reproduction on microfilms or in any other physical way, and transmission or information storage and retrieval, electronic adaptation, computer software, or by similar or dissimilar methodology now known or hereafter developed.
The use of general descriptive names, registered names, trademarks, service marks, etc. in this publication does not imply, even in the absence of a specific statement, that such names are exempt from the relevant protective laws and regulations and therefore free for general use.
The publisher, the authors, and the editors are safe to assume that the advice and information in this book are believed to be true and accurate at the date of publication. Neither the publisher nor the authors or the editors give a warranty, expressed or implied, with respect to the material contained herein or for any errors or omissions that may have been made. The publisher remains neutral with regard to jurisdictional claims in published maps and institutional affiliations.

This Springer imprint is published by the registered company Springer Nature Switzerland AG
The registered company address is: Gewerbestrasse 11, 6330 Cham, Switzerland

Paper in this product is recyclable.

Foreword

It is my pleasure to contribute a foreword to this volume on *Building Your Academic Research Digital Identity*, authored and edited by Kyle Downey and Peggy Dreker. As an author/editor of a number of books and dozens of articles on some abstract topics for library and information science field—like the relationship of libraries to democracy, I have benefitted from the networks and tools described in this volume, albeit inadvertently much of the time. With Peggy and Kyle, I am also at Seton Hall as Dean of University Libraries and Associate Provost for Research and Innovation. As an academic administrator I have copious opportunities to investigate candidates' and researchers' profiles and how they present themselves because it makes a difference and colors how one views credentials and research. Like it or not, such information frames one's work. What follows are a few observations from a few decades of looking at applications, dossiers, CVs, social media and web profiles, and so on.

First, less is more. By this I mean personal information. An "about me" profile on an academic institution's web page from years ago is seared in my memory: "Pat still misses the atmosphere of Cupcake and *alma mater*, the University of Cupcake, where community, local music, and potlucks with friends abounded. To get away from the rigors of academic life, the soft sand of the beaches 2 h away beckoned, particularly lovely on fall evenings." Fictionalized, it is a real example, and current ones are not hard to find on LinkedIn, social media, or other sources: family and relationship statuses, a penchant for Buffalo Wild Wings, Lego block arrangements satirizing academia, and complaints about anonymous reviewers are all real examples. If you absolutely must, a wall of separation between your work/scholarship and such ... shall we say expressions of identity is essential.

Second, more is more. If I must hunt down information that another academic might want and that should be reasonably public—undergraduate degree, graduate degree(s), the places and field(s) of study—then my antennae are up. Questions are raised: why is this so hard to find? Others follow: is there study and expertise behind this scholarship, or not? What else has the author published of relevance? And so on. I don't mean that these must be thrust in the face, but scholarship and academics run on intellectual *bone fides* and trust, and these are the first (albeit highly imperfect, it will be said here) elements of them.

Third, don't bother protesting that the rules don't uniformly apply: they don't. There is a pecking order. I know that the Harvard historian and *New Yorker* contributor Jill Lepore has three sons because Professor Lepore is famous. Likewise, Paul Krugman, Imani Perry, or Danielle Allen—all scholars I (lightly) follow. We're not them. Get over it.

Finally, assuming your scholarship has merit, this works. In recent e-mails with a now-retired scholar, they were embarrassed to admit that they didn't really know how to expose their work, always just publishing where they did and assuming people would find it, if interested. The lack of coordinated information about them and easier access to their scholarship showed: this person's Google Scholar profile has half-to-one-third fewer citations than contemporaries—recently retired scholars working in the same vein, in the same field, of a similar high quality of publication.

So *nota bene* the perspectives and advice you encounter in this volume—and where/who it comes from: in a plug for my own field, librarians know and understand the plumbing—the inner workings—of these scholarly ecosystems, perhaps more than you do. Use their skills.

University Libraries, Seton Hall University   John Buschman
South Orange, NJ, USA

He is the author of many publications including Libraries, classrooms, and the interests of democracy: Marking the limits of neoliberalism (2012, Rowman & Littlefield/Scarecrow Press). Google Scholar profile: https://tinyurl.com/JEBSHU.

Foreword

Mr. Kyle Downey and Ms. Peggy Dreker have fashioned an important book for academic researchers seeking to make connections and create an online presence in the modern digital age.

Research has never been more of a team sport. The days of research siloes with isolated investigators working only with their own staff are long gone. It is a time of "open" laboratories where research groups share not only space and equipment—but expertise. The move has been towards research enterprises serving as intellectual incubators—with shared resources, knowledge, and skill. Researchers must connect in the exceedingly complex digital world that exists today. That is where *Building Your Academic Research Digital Identity: A Step-Wise Guide to Cultivating Your Academic Research Career Online* comes in—it provides a road map to navigate this space. The book beautifully articulates digital tools that may be best employed to facilitate networking, collaboration, and creating an online presence that accurately describes one's professional identity and maximizes one's research visibility. This is important information and a must read for those engaged in trying to establish such identities.

I have been a biomedical researcher in a university/medical school setting since entering graduate school in 1987. I found the academic scholar track to be challenging—while at the same time tremendously rewarding. I supported my work through extramural funding, worked tirelessly to move research initiatives forward, and taught professional and graduate students all along the way. The academic researcher's life is one that I have embraced and am proud to have been a part of. To grow a regional, national, and ultimately international presence/reputation, I needed to have my research considered in the best light far and wide—requiring publications, presentations, and—where possible—collaborations. This approach has worked for many investigators over the years—but times have changed.

Importantly, this book offers a how-to guide for researchers, faculty, and students, to develop strategies designed to burnish their academic brand, and craft the best possible research persona in the modern age. The strategies and insights offered are unique in many ways—there are not many collated sources available that address this extremely important topic. I enthusiastically endorse this timely and essential guide for academic researchers and related educators.

Department of Medical Sciences   Stanley R. Terlecky
Hackensack Meridian School of Medicine,
NJ, USA

Acknowledgments

First and foremost, I want to thank my coauthor and editor Peggy Dreker for her expertise and commitment to this project. I am truly grateful for her getting this project off the ground and I am honored to have had the opportunity to collaborate with someone as dedicated and knowledgeable as her. To my wife, Kristen, without your support and encouragement this would have been more difficult to accomplish. To my son Nathaniel, I hope this inspires you to challenge yourself and always express your individuality without compromise. And lastly, to my parents, who have always inspired me to publish.—*Kyle James Downey*

Words cannot express my gratitude to my coeditor/author Kyle Downey for his patience and invaluable contributions to this project. His knowledge and expertise made for the perfect writing partner. Thanks to my family who expressed doubts about my consistent refrain, "I can't go I'm busy." To the person who continually said you should write a book, well I did!—*Peggy Rush Dreker*

Christopher P. Duffy, MLIS, AHIP, the Associate Dean and founding Director for the Interprofessional Health Sciences Library, serving Seton Hall University and Hackensack-Meridian School of Medicine, for his leadership, encouragement, guidance, and patience.

We want to thank all the chapter authors for bringing their expertise to the table. Their commitment to this project demonstrates their dedication to the profession.

Dr. John Bushman, Associate Provost for Research and Innovation and Dean of University Libraries at Seton Hall University, and Dr. Stanley Terlecky, Professor and Chair, Department of Medical Sciences at Hackensack Meridian School of Medicine, for their leadership, guidance, and contributions to this book.

We would like to extend a thank you to Seton Hall University and Hackensack Meridian School of Medicine communities for all their support. Their encouragement allows us to share this information with our students and faculty.

We hope this book will prove helpful to our fellow colleagues and researchers in understanding the importance of research and digital identity.

Contents

1 **Why Create a Digital Identity?** 1
   Kyle James Downey and Margaret Rush Dreker

2 **Why Manage Your Digital Identity Online** 9
   Margaret Rush Dreker

3 **Managing Your Research Identity and the Role of the Librarian** 23
   Gerald Shea

4 **Managing Your Digital Research Identity with ORCID** 35
   Yingting Zhang

5 **Tools for Managing Your Digital Research Identity** 51
   Layal Hneiny

6 **Author Metrics** 69
   Kyle James Downey

7 **Additional Measures to Establish Your Digital Identity** 85
   Plato Smith

8 **Building Your Digital Presence on Social Media** 101
   Matthew Bridgeman

9 **Risks, Privacy, and Harassment** 127
   Margaret Rush Dreker

10 **Mapping Out Your Digital Presence** 141
   Kyle James Downey and Margaret Rush Dreker

Correction to: Tools for Managing Your Digital Research Identity C1
   Layal Hneiny

Index 151

Editors and Contributors

About the Editors

Margaret Rush Dreker, (Peggy Dreker), MPA, MLS, is a Medical Librarian at the Interprofessional Health Sciences Library at Hackensack Meridian School of Medicine in Nutley, NJ. Peggy is an Instructor in the Department of Medical Sciences at Hackensack Meridian School of Medicine and a Lecturer at Seton Hall University in South Orange, NJ. Peggy received an MPA from New York University and MLS from Rutgers University. Peggy spent 20 years at the George F. Smith Library of the Health Sciences at Rutgers University in Newark, NJ. In her work, Peggy provides research support services to the students, faculty, and researchers at HMSOM. The services she provides include teaching in the Information Mastery curriculum, support of the Problem Based Learning curriculum, literature searching, citation management, research metrics and impact, systematic reviews, scholarly publishing in addition to performing health sciences information services responsibilities.

Kyle James Downey, MLIS, is Health Sciences and Nursing Librarian at Seton Hall University. He holds a Master of Library and Information Sciences from Rutgers University and a bachelor's degree in history from Rutgers University. Working at the Interprofessional Health Sciences Library in Nutley, NJ, Kyle provides library research support to students, faculty, and administration for the College of Nursing and the School of Health and Medical Sciences. Kyle provides instructional support to undergraduate, graduate, and postgraduate students as well as research support in the form of literature searching assistance, citation, and data management. Prior to working in academia, Kyle worked as a Medical Librarian at Robert Wood Johnson University Hospital, Somerset, where he provided library services to physicians, nurses, and residents. Kyle's research interests include research and citation impact, evidence-based searching skills, and library curriculum development. He has given presentations at the Medical Library Association (MLA) and has recently published an article on the integration and assessment of library instruction in a graduate Physical Therapy curriculum. Kyle continues to find ways to integrate library instruction in order to help students develop the fundamental skills that will be needed once they graduate and find work.

Contributors

Matthew Bridgeman is an Education and Instruction Librarian at the Robert Wood Johnson Library of the Health Sciences at Rutgers University. He serves the Ernest Mario School of Pharmacy and the Physician Assistant program. His specializations include systematic reviews, data visualization, instruction, and outreach. In addition, he is a member of the Diversity, Equity, and Inclusion Committee and social media Coordinator team at Rutgers University Libraries where he manages the Health Sciences Libraries Instagram account.

Layal Hneiny In 2007 as a graduate of Chemistry, Layal taught Chemistry in SABIS in Abu Dhabi and AlAin. She first joined the American University of Beirut (AUB) University Libraries—Jafet Library in 2008 as a Library Assistant in the Serials & Electronic Resources Department. In 2014, she joined Saab Medical Library (SML) as the assistant to the medical librarian, after attaining her MPH-HMP from AUB. She was then promoted to Medical & Health Sciences Librarian, in 2018, after earning her MLIS degree from the University of Pittsburgh. Hneiny possesses over a decade of experience at the University Libraries at AUB assisting physicians, faculty, and students. She instructs researchers on topics such as where to publish and how to increase their research impact. She has been a contributor to many health-related courses and programs at the AUB, including the Research Personnel Program (RPP) and the Fellowship and Residency Research Program (FRRP). She teaches classes on health information literacy to graduates and Ph.D. students at the medical school and Med 1 students. Layal is a Clinical Research Librarian at the University Miami - Florida.

Gerard Shea is a tenured librarian at Seton Hall University. He serves as the subject liaison to the College of Communication and the Arts and is also a co-liaison for the English Department and College of Education and Human Services. Shea received an MLS from Pratt Institute and an MA in Special Education from New Jersey City University.

His research interests include information literacy, autism spectrum disorder, and scholarly communication. His publications include four articles in peer-reviewed journals, and he was the lead author for two articles on library services for autistic college students, *Academic Libraries and Autism Spectrum Order: What Do We Know?* and *A Survey of Library Services for Autistic Students*, which were published by *The Journal of Academic Librarianship*. In 2020, Shea co-wrote an article on the circulation of print books at Walsh Library, *Read In or Check Out: A Four-Year Analysis of Circulation and In-House Use of Print Books*, which was also published in *The Journal of Academic Librarianship*. The article examines the decline in print book circulation at Walsh Library and at academic libraries in general. He additionally co-wrote the article, *Leveraging Undergraduate Federal Work Study Student Skill Sets to Support an R2 University Libraries' Research Data Services*, which was published in *College & Undergraduate Libraries* in 2021. The article discusses approaches to establishing a research data services (RDS) program at an R2 institution with a limited budget.

In his leisure time, he enjoys spending time with his family and Sheeba, their puppy, and Pixie, their Chinchilla. He also enjoys playing basketball with his two sons, Jake and Dillon. And he passionately follows the Seton Hall basketball team and the New York Yankees.

Plato L. Smith II, Ph.D. is the Data Management Librarian and an Associate University Librarian at the University of Florida in Gainesville, Florida, USA. He has over 15 years of experience in academic research libraries. Dr. Smith assists in the development of socio-technical (people, policies, technologies) relationships with diverse stakeholders and chairs the Data Management and Curation Working Group (DMCWG) at the University of Florida (UF). Prior to joining UF in 2016, he completed the 2014–2016 CLIR Postdoctoral Fellowship Program in Data Curation at the University of New Mexico. He received his doctorate in the field of Information Science from the School of Information within the College of Communication and Information at Florida State

University, Florida's iSchool. He has experience in digital libraries and data management, and his Master of Science is from the Graduate School of Library and Information Sciences at North Carolina Central University. He specializes in the study of data management and curation and its interdisciplinary synergistic implications across multiple communities of practice. His current research focuses on (a) exploring data management and curation practices of researchers across disciplines, (b) sharing faculty research data, and (c) data repositories.

Yingting Zhang is the Research Services Librarian at the Robert Wood Johnson (RWJ) Library of the Health Sciences and Adjunct Assistant Professor in the Department of Medicine of the RWJ Medical School at Rutgers University. In her work, Yingting provides research support services to researchers, faculty, students, and staff at Rutgers Biomedical and Health Sciences (RBHS) and beyond. The services she provides include but not limited to compliance with NIH Public Access Policy and NIH Data Management and Sharing Policy, Developing NIH Biosketches, Creating and Connecting ORCID iD to Rutgers NetID, citation management, research metrics and impact, scholarly publishing, systematic reviews in addition to teaching and performing health sciences information services. Yingting served on the ORCID Implementation Team at Rutgers and assists researchers with questions on ORCID. She was recognized for her outreach work by the ORCID US Community in 2022. Yingting is a distinguished member of the Medical Library Association's Academy of Health Information Professionals. She serves on the Rutgers Health Sciences Institutional Review Board (IRB) and is a member of the Executive IRB.

Abbreviations

AHRQ	Agency of Healthcare Research Quality
AI	Amnesty International
AIF	Author Impact Factor
AMA	American Medical Association
API	Application Programming Interfaces
ASNS	Academic Social Networking Sites
BMIC	Biomedical Informatics Coordinating Committee
CC	Code of Conduct
CDC	Centers for Disease Control and Prevention
CLIR	Council on Library and Information Services
CRIS	Current Research Information System
CV	Curriculum Vitae
DMP	Data Management and Sharing Plans
DOI	Digital Object Identifier
E-Index	Author Level Metric
GAP	Global Access Program
G-Index	Author Level Metric
GS	Google Scholar
HAL	Hyper Articles EN LIGNE
H-index	Hirsch Index
HMSOM	Hackensack Meridian School of Medicine
IASSIST	International Association for Social Science Information Services and Technology
IATUL	International Association of University Libraries
ICGL	International Conference on Gray Literature
ICMJE	International Committee of Medical Journal Editors
ICPSR	Inter-University Consortium for Political and Social Research
IDCC	International Digital Curation Conference
IHS	Interprofessional Health Sciences
IMLS	Institute of Museum and Library Services
IOP	Institute of Physics

IR	Institutional Repository
JaLC	Japan Link Center
NASA	National Aeronautics and Space Administration
NCBI	National Center Biology Technology Information
NIH	National Institute of Health
NLM	National Library of Medicine
NSF	National Science Foundation
NSPM	National Security Presidential Memoranda
OA	Open Access
ORCID	Open Researcher and Contributor ID
OSTP	Office of Science and Technology Policy
PDI	Persistent Digital Identifier
PLOS	Public Library of Science
PMID	PubMed Identifier
RG	ResearchGate
RIMS	Research Information Management System
ROR	Research Organization Registry
SciENcv	Science Experts Network Curriculum Vitae
SHU	Seton Hall University
STEM	Science Technology Engineering Mathematics
UF	University of Florida
UFIRST	University of Florida Integrated Research Support Tool
UH	University of Houston
UMN	University of Minnesota
UNESCO	United Nations Educational, Scientific and Cultural Organization
URL	Uniform Resource Locator
WoS	Web of Science

Chapter 1
Why Create a Digital Identity?

Kyle James Downey and Margaret Rush Dreker

Identity and Digital Identity

Identity is "the unique set of characteristics that can be used to identify a person as themself and no one else. The word can be used in different ways in different contexts. On a personal level, identity often refers to a person's sense of self, meaning how they view themself as compared to other people". [1, 2] Personality traits, abilities, likes and dislikes, your belief system or moral code, and the things that motivate you—these all contribute to self-image or your unique identity as a person.

Your professional identity is professional self-concept of an individual grounded in attributes, beliefs, motives, values, and experiences, "the attitudes, values, knowledge, beliefs and skills shared with others within a professional group" [3]. The development of professional identity has been defined as a continuous process that is influenced by several factors including experiences in practice and professional socialization [4]. A significant amount of this development occurs during an individual's time completing their education. Professional identity is considered a dynamic phenomenon, which continues to evolve from university study into a health professionals' work life [5].

Digital identity is information used by computer systems to represent an external agent—a person, organization, application, or device. Digital identities allow access to services provided with computers to be automated and make it possible for computers to mediate relationships [2]. The use of the term digital identity is so broad

K. J. Downey (✉)
College of Nursing & School of Health and Medical Sciences Librarian, Seton Hall University, Nutley, NJ, USA
e-mail: kyle.downey@shu.edu

M. R. Dreker
Hackensack Meridian School of Medicine, Nutley, NJ, USA
e-mail: margaret.dreker@hmhn.org

© The Author(s), under exclusive license to Springer Nature Switzerland AG 2023
M. R. Dreker, K. J. Downey (eds.), *Building Your Academic Research Digital Identity*, https://doi.org/10.1007/978-3-031-50317-7_1

any digital activity of an individual's online history is referred to as a "digital identity." There are many unique identifiers that can make up a digital identity such as name, age, gender, personal information, affiliation, education, research interest, and more.

Your digital identity is any trail that you left in your life that is now online. In academics a digital identity promotes and defines a person's knowledge, and research in their respective fields. A digital identity is a representation of a person's real self, online. Your digital identity is completed with all the online information and data specifically about you as an individual.

Which Platform Do I Use to Establish My Digital Identity?

It is becoming harder to understand and to manage all the online platforms available. How do you choose which platforms to establish your digital profile? Are there rules and regulations on how to use a platform? Has your institution implemented social media guidelines? Does your field of research have professional standards or ethics when it comes to social media?

Building your digital identity as a researcher can be an effective way to publicize your work among your peers. Developing these skills can lay out a path to professional advancement in hiring, promotion, and tenure. It can help build networks which can lead to collaborations, increased research, and grants. Having a well-managed identity helps engage with the public disseminating of your knowledge to students, public, and the media. It can also help prevent misinformation.

The Internet was designed without any guidelines or rules identifying who the experts are in a particular field. Anyone online could be viewed as an expert. There is not a license to prove who you are and that you have the authority to speak about a topic.

You can use social media platforms and Academic Social Networking Sites or ASNS to promote your new publications or your scheduled talk at a professional conference. You can increase your engagement and following on social media by sharing other relevant content that is of interest to your audience. Digital platforms have wide abilities to reach audiences all over the world which is why you want to pay close attention to how you are portrayed on each platform.

Academic Social Networks Sites (ASNS) have changed how information is shared and communicated. Full papers are being shared along with teaching materials and general discussions. Those hoping for publications are now using ASNS and preprint servers to offer their research to the public instead of exploring the traditional publication route. Management of your online profile on whichever network you choose, becomes essential. A researcher can present their professional experiences, ideas, and capabilities, including the number of citations and downloads of his/her articles and promoting an online identity. This also allows for networking opportunities and potential collaborations. Many platforms have built in email components or text messaging systems along with storge for publications and collaborations. Online ASNS also provide author metrics and measurement to record research impact.

Choosing the social media platforms your colleagues are using, or which platforms your professional organizations are using, is a smart thing to do before setting up your digital profiles. You can establish different profiles or identities on each platform. You can make information public and keep some private. It is all up to you.

Writing for a Digital Platform

Be aware of the tone and permanence of your voice on social media. Think carefully about how personal you are willing to be, the tones of your posts and the type of language you convey. Be sure the manner and the content of your social media posts are consistent and remain a reflection of your work and not you personally.

Don't post for the sake of it! Try to plan ahead. Schedule a weekly or monthly social media activity to promote the relevant outcomes of your research. Take time to prepare your interaction. Be sure your content is always kept up to date. Prepare by writing a draft post or blog entry, curate materials for sharing, find users you want to tag and seek out an existing hashtag that will improve the reach of your social media posts.

Academics and researchers use digital platforms for many reasons; self-promotion, to belong to a professional community, to acquire professional knowledge, and to interact with other professionals [6]. As you build your network, you must remember that your interaction is as important for establishing your digital identity and profile as any information about you. Networking is about forming relationships with others. It is important to establish online communication practices that project a thoughtful, positive, and professional individual.

Public Writing

It's important to target your audience when writing for the web. By knowing who you are writing for, you can write at a level that will be meaningful for them. Public writing is writing with a public purpose. That public purpose might be to inform, persuade, or create change. Public writing is typically crafted for a particular audience, and it translates complex ideas and research into succinct prose. Public writing is writing for impact [7].

Writing for the Web

Social media is the new public forum. Writing on social media is a well-established area with common best practices. Be sure to consider the following as you write any type of online content:

1. Use the words your users use. By using keywords that your users use, you will help them understand the content and will help optimize it for search engines.
2. Chunk your content. Chunking makes your content more scannable by breaking it into manageable sections.
3. Front-load the important information. Use the journalism model of the "inverted pyramid." Start with the content that is most important to your audience, and then provide additional details.
4. Use active voice. "The board proposed the legislation" not "The regulation was proposed by the board."
5. Use short sentences and paragraphs. The ideal standard is no more than 20 words per sentence, five sentences per paragraph. Use dashes instead of semi-colons or, better yet, break the sentence into two.
6. Use bullets and numbered lists. Don't limit yourself to using this for long lists—one sentence and two bullets is easier to read than three sentences.
7. Use clear headlines and subheads. Questions are particularly effective.
8. Use images, diagrams, or multimedia to visually reinforce ideas in the text. Make sure all visuals and media are accessible [7].

Before establishing your digital identity on any platform, seek out your institutional guidance regarding the use of social networks and social media. Be sure your identity is professional. Read the harassment policies of each platform before you establish your profile.

In academia many think that a person's record of success and professional recognition is just publications and research. That is partially true but that is not all one will be evaluated on. Professional networking through a positive and well thought out personal digital identity will help establish credibility and reputation with the community of academics and researchers. It will also help you expand outside your opportunities in the world beyond academia [8].

Organization of This Book

We have designed this book for academics and researchers to communicate scholarly work in a productive and time efficient manner. This book aims to help you be strategic and smart in how you navigate academic and social media platforms and harness its immense benefits.

This book will discuss topics which will help you establish and maintain your digital identity including the management of your digital footprint.

The broad topic on why it is important to manage your digital identity will be discussed in Chapter 2. This chapter will offer guidance on the importance of developing your personal identity which is linked to your professional reputation. Therefore, in this book we will explore the interaction between a user (a human), their identity information stored and maintained digitally. In other words, we will be dealing exclusively with personal identity management.

The digital transformation of the research forces the researchers to open and maintain different digital profiles. That can be done strategically, selecting the mandatory platforms and choosing those that are relevant.

Chapter 3 will explore the role of the academic librarian in teaching digital identity. Academic librarians actively contribute to the scholarly productivity at their respective universities and organizations. This chapter elaborates on how new technologies and metrics for measuring scholarly impact are changing the academic environment. Academic librarians have the role of teaching these scholarly tools to their faculty and students so that they can establish a research presence in their disciplines. This includes educating them on topics, such as author rights, self-archiving, and alternative metrics.

Librarians want to encourage their colleagues to establish or increase their scholarly presence in this complicated and ever-changing world. With so many new metrics, platforms, and tools available, librarians are there to assist those who may be concerned about adapting to these new methods and ideas. In the world of research, the librarian is a key resource in establishing or increasing one's scholarly presence.

Chapter 4 will introduce tools to manage your digital identity such as Open Researcher and Contributor ID or ORCID. By establishing a digital identity, a person can increase the impact of their research by building an online presence. This will make it easy for researchers, scholars, students, organizations, funding bodies, and other knowledge users to find them and their work.

A digital identity helps ensure that research is available to the widest possible audience and improves its discoverability and dissemination. One digital platform available to build an online presence, and distinguish yourself, your research, and professional activities is by claiming an ORCiD. ORCID is an open, non-profit, international registry of unique and persistent identifiers for individual researchers. It is the preferred way to link identifiers with researchers' outputs and activities.

Chapter 5 will review the growth of digital platforms and the wide range of tools available to researchers that will help manage one's digital identity. Understanding what these tools do will allow researchers to measure their reach, influence, and establish collaborative opportunities with others.

Platforms that will be discussed include LinkedIn, PubMed Profile, and Doximity. Subscription-based tools such as Scopus-Author ID and Web of Science-ResearcherID will also be examined. Other tools showcase traditional and alternative author metrics will also be reviewed.

Chapter 6 will discuss how research impact affects the use, or influence of research findings [9]. An author's impact is measured by using the number of times his/her a publication is cited by other researchers (also known as citation metrics). Citation metrics are used to determine the impact and productivity of a researcher.

The most common author metric, that uses a citation metric, is the h-index. This calculation combines two variables to attribute impact to a researcher: the number of publications, and the number of citations. The h-index, the most common author metric, is often used as a "yardstick" to measure and compare researchers and scholars.

To combat challenges related to the h-index, scholars have created additional author metrics. However, these metrics also use the same citation data as the h-index and as a consequence also suffer from some of the same issues.

This chapter will also review the topic of alternative metrics (or altmetrics). Altmetrics are metrics that monitor and measure the reach and impact of scholarship online interactions, complementing the traditional measures of academic success using citation impact. Traditional measures of citation only represent one type of impact and does not reflect the changing scholarly horizon that has moved beyond print. Altmetrics tracks the online interaction with research outputs such as articles, datasets, tools, social media, videos, etc. as a way of measuring research impact and reach.

There are added measures to establish a digital identity that will be discussed in Chapter 7. Developing a professional website that chronicles your academic career achievements is an added measure in establishing a digital identity. This chapter will explore resources that will increase one's digital presence with discussions on topics such as: Open Access (OA), data repositories, ORCiDs, and others. Headings included on one's website should contain Research, Scholarly Works, Awards, Teaching, Service, and Curriculum Vitae.

Maintaining and curating a personal professional website requires a serious time commitment. There are tools that are available to users to streamline the process. The author uses a case study on modeling his own personal professional website.

Chapter 8 will delve into social media and its uses in establishing a digital identity. Social media includes online platforms that enable people to interact and communicate with each other. Through these virtual networks, social media facilitates the creation and sharing of content, thoughts, and information. The use of social media has changed in the past years, and it is no longer a platform to be just "social" but a way to share and disseminate academic materials and research.

In this chapter social media will be discussed as a tool of presenting one's research presence. Researchers and academics use these platforms to discuss new research ideas, to identify collaborators, to communicate with colleagues around the world and to disseminate findings.

Although there are benefits of digital platforms there are challenges of maintaining your digital identity that will be discussed in Chapter 9. There are many platforms available to academics to form a digital identity. With the increased use of ASNS and social media, comes concerns about privacy and security. Security issues that academics face include harassment, identity theft, plagiarism, and more.

These concerns revolve around the main issue of "professional reputation." Any misuse of social media or digital platforms can cause irreputable harm to the researcher, their institution and destroy a career. This chapter will examine these issues and provide some best practices for future use.

Summary

In this book you will learn about the various tools, platforms, and metrics that will help establish your digital profile. Whether you are new in the field of research and publishing or you have a well-established portfolio of written literature, this book will provide guidance in establishing your digital research presence. You will also discover new ways to engage with and use academic social networking and social media platforms to your advantage.

References

1. Marshall K. How to curate your digital identity as an academic. The Chronicle of Higher Education. January 5, 2015. https://www.chronicle.com/article/how-to-curate-your-digital-identity-as-an-academic/. Accessed 3 Feb 2023.
2. Identity. 2023. https://www.dictionary.com. Accessed 2 Feb 2023.
3. Adams K, Hean S, Sturgis P, Clark JM. Investigating the factors influencing professional identity of first-year health and social care students. Learn Health Soc Care. 2006;5(2):55–68. https://doi.org/10.1111/j.1473-6861.2006.00119.x.
4. Ashby SE, Adler J, Herbert L. An exploratory international study into occupational therapy students' perceptions of professional identity. Aust Occup Ther J. 2016;63(4):233–43. https://doi.org/10.1111/1440-1630.12271.
5. Trede F, Macklin R, Bridges D. Professional identity development: a review of the higher education literature. Stud High Educ. 2012;37(3):365–84. https://doi.org/10.1080/03075079.2010.521237.
6. Meishar-Tal H, Pieterse E. Why do academics use academic social networking sites? Int Rev Res Open Distribut Learn. 2017;18(1) https://doi.org/10.19173/irrodl.v18i1.2643.
7. Hattwig D, Shayne J, Berger A, Wyly K. Public writing guide. 2022. Licensed under Creative Commons Attribution 4.0 International License. https://guides.lib.uw.edu/bothell/publicwriting/writingfortheweb. Accessed 2 Mar 2023.
8. Crash Override Network. What to do if your employee is being targeted by online abuse. http://www.crashoverridenetwork.com/employers.html. Accessed 21 Jan 2023.
9. Penfield T, Baker MJ, Scoble R, Wykes MC. Assessment, evaluations, and definitions of research impact: a review. Res Eval. 2013;23(1):21–32. https://doi.org/10.1093/reseval/rvt021.

Chapter 2
Why Manage Your Digital Identity Online

Margaret Rush Dreker

Introduction

Digital technologies, and the immediacy, visibility, and connectedness they imply, have changed the way we communicate and present ourselves. Social media offers new opportunities for self-presentation, impression management, self-promotion, and identity performance. In the academic world, there has also been a shift in the ways in which scholars present themselves publicly. They are increasingly turning to online spaces (e.g., faculty webpages, social networking sites, academic blogs) to create an online persona, develop professional identities, and claim their place within their disciplinary community and even outside academia [1].

Academic Social Networks Sites

Generic social media sites, such as Facebook, Instagram, and Twitter or X, are available to everyone to use as they see fit. The Academic Social Networks Sites (ASNS) which are geared toward a specific group of professionals, started popping up in the early 2000s. Academic Social Networks Sites (ASNS) are similar to social networking sites but are designed for the academic community. These online platforms allow researchers, professors, and scientists to develop an individual profile and connect with other like-minded people, while also allowing them to share academic-related content. Many of these tools are typically free to use.

ASNS can be divided into two categories as outlined by Jordon:

M. R. Dreker (✉)
Hackensack Meridian School of Medicine, Nutley, NJ, USA
e-mail: Margaret.dreker@hmhn.org

© The Author(s), under exclusive license to Springer Nature
Switzerland AG 2023
M. R. Dreker, K. J. Downey (eds.), *Building Your Academic Research Digital Identity*, https://doi.org/10.1007/978-3-031-50317-7_2

- Those that have been developed primarily to facilitate profile creation and connect (analogous to Facebook; examples include Academia.edu and ResearchGate).
- Those with a primary focus on posting and sharing academic-related content and have subsequently added social networking capabilities (such as Mendeley) [2].

Some other benefits of the ASNS include academic openness, sharing and dissemination, self-promotion and online persona management, research and collaboration, teaching, impact measurement, documents management, and professional support.

Why Publish

In the world of academia, the motto of "publish or perish" has haunted the hallways for hundreds of years. There is even more pressure on researchers to publish for multiple reasons including promotion, tenure, grant money, and more. The purpose of publishing original research studies is to disseminate the results of experiments to inform the audience about a new concept or about advances in a technology or scientific field. Publishing provides a communication channel for researchers within a field, a repository of a researcher's efforts, and a recognition measurement or impact factor for researchers and institutions alike. ASNS assist in many of these steps on a researcher's career path. ASNS can act as a professional self-archiving platform for researchers to upload, store, and disseminate their work. These international platforms can allow further dissemination of work, which can lead to higher author metrics and impact factors which can advance a researcher's career. It is vital that the work is attributed to the correct author.

Why Authorship Matters?

Authorship confers credit and has important academic, social, and financial implications. Authorship also implies responsibility and accountability for published work. The following recommendations are intended to ensure that contributors who have made substantive intellectual contributions to a paper are given credit as authors, but also that contributors credited as authors understand their role in taking responsibility and being accountable for what is published [3].

The International Committee of Medical Journal Editors (ICMJE) recommends that authorship be based on the following criteria:

- Substantial contributions to the conception or design of the work; or the acquisition, analysis, or interpretation of data for the work; and
- Drafting the work or revising it critically for important intellectual content; and
- Final approval of the version to be published; and

– Agreement to be accountable for all aspects of the work in ensuring that questions related to the accuracy or integrity of any part of the work are appropriately investigated and resolved [3]

What's in a Name?

Many researchers have names shared with others and are faced with an ongoing challenge to distinguish their research from that of others. Academics and researchers change their affiliated organizations as they move on to different stages of their careers. Some authors have the added complication of changing their name through marriage (or divorce), once or more during their professional careers. Ideally, they need to be able to attach their own identity easily and uniquely to all their own research outputs including original articles, datasets, blogs, opinion pieces, scholarly letters, patents, and grant applications [4].

Women still predominantly make decisions regarding martial name changes. In science, technology, engineering, and mathematics (STEM) fields, as the proportion of female researchers rises, more women are considering the potential effects of martial name change on their careers. The stakes are high, as relationship status and name discrimination contribute to gender and racial inequities in faculty hiring. Names can also reveal racial, ethnic, religious, or cultural aspects of a person's identity that one may not want to share in their professional lives [5].

One of the main challenges for tracking research output and publications is name ambiguity. In recent years, research productivity has grown tremendously, making it difficult to distinguish who the author of a particular work may be due to identical or similar names or name changes [6]. The growth of a single name change system through using an Open Researcher and Contributor ID or ORCID iDs would also support the transgender researchers community and those considering marital names change [5] Creating a digital profile or digital identifier could assist with any name ambiguity.

Digital Profile

A digital profile is the sum content about a person that appears on the Internet [7]. A digital profile or digital identity is a mix of personal and professional information shared on different social media platforms and the Internet. The information could have been posted personally or by others. Biographical information could have been provided when you presented at an annual conference. Background information could have been provided by you on LinkedIn or even on your organizational web site on the page titled "About Us" or "Meet Our Staff" (Fig. 2.1). The information is out there! It is your responsibility to see that the information is curated and is accurate.

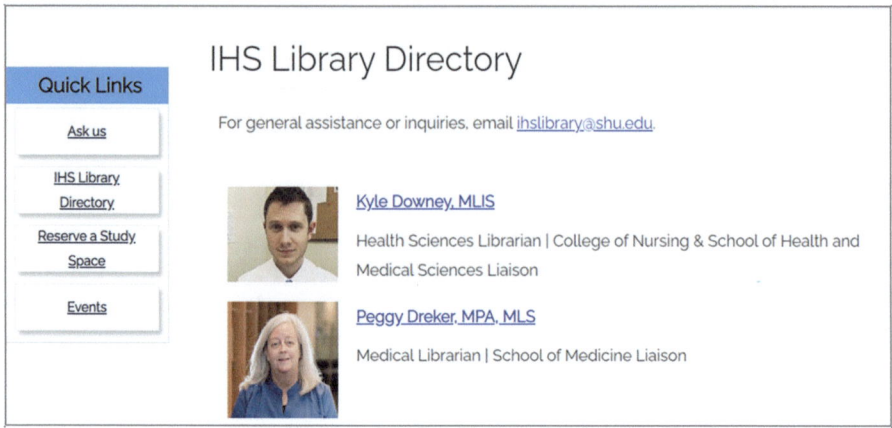

Fig. 2.1 IHS Library Staff Directory. https://library.shu.edu/ihs/pages/directory

Who Are You in the Digital Universe?

The best way to see what is currently existing in your digital profile is to enter your name, and any variations, into a search engine. Search engines index social media platforms so if you have a Facebook account it will come up when you search on your name. This will also occur with your LinkedIn profile and most social media accounts.

Select the Images tab in the search engine. Do any personal photos appear in the search results of your name? Is this OK with you? Is a professional headshot found in the image search? Is your institutional profile visible and current? Do you appear at the top of the search results?

When I searched my name, Margaret Dreker or Dreker MR, it provided results from my Google Scholar profile, my LinkedIn profile, my Research Gate profile, a few articles indexed in PubMed, and my professional organizations home page (Fig. 2.2).

The search also links me to a German Trash Metal band named "Dreker" (not me) and to a 1999 Congressional Testimony before the Subcommittee on Health and Environment (which was me). Some of the information is correct and other information is not accurate or what I would like associated with my "professional profile."

In the world of academics and research, reputation is everything. Employment, promotion, tenure, dissemination of research, and collaboration all depend on reputation. That reputation is now available for everyone to see so it is vital to be sure the information and opinions are accurate and attributed to the correct person.

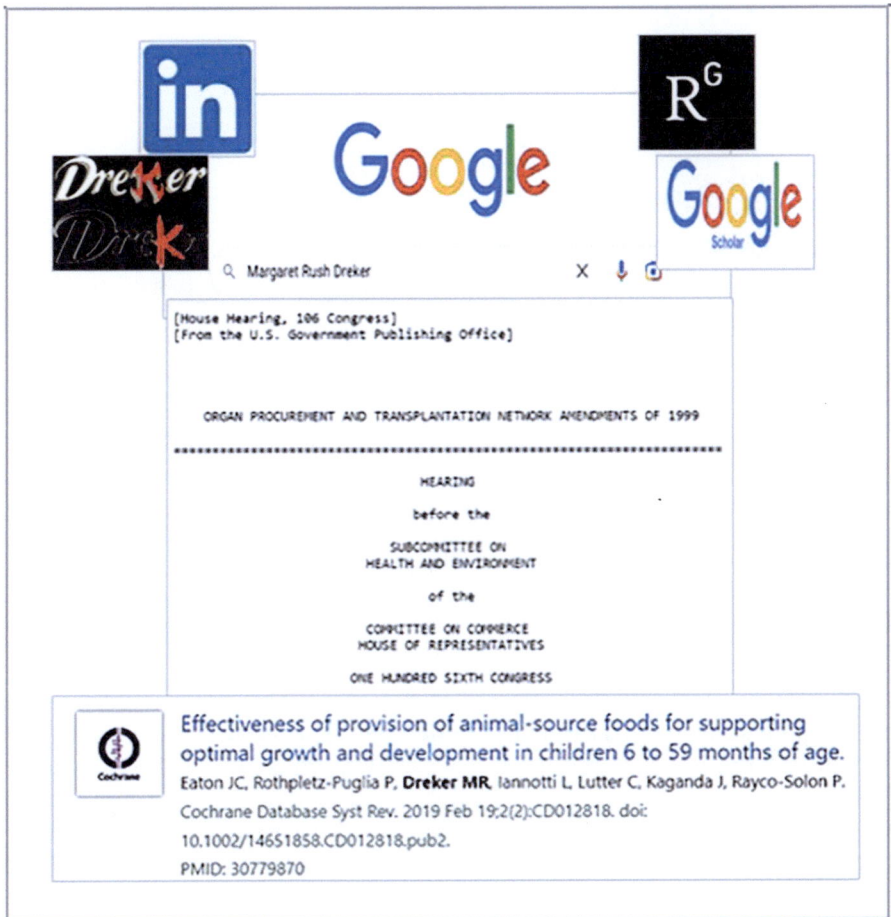

Fig. 2.2 Google search on Margaret Rush Dreker

Measure Your Research Impact Online

Bibliometrics and Altmetrics provide measures of the attention your research is getting (see Chapter 6). Bibliometrics track and measure citations across scholarly publications, while altmetrics represents the wider attention that your publications are getting beyond the academic community in social media and mainstream media. Many tenure and promotion committees now look at altmetrics scores to see how you are using social media platforms to disseminate your research (Fig. 2.3).

10 Tips to Improve Your Visibility and Your Research

1. Create profiles on sites that rank highly in search results.
2. Manage your name by getting an ORCID identifier.
3. Make your web address easy to find.
4. Create a single home for your online presence.
5. Link your online profiles together.
6. Write guest posts on other people's blogs to gain more visibility.
7. Decide if you will have a personal or a professional digital profile.
8. Use appropriate images online.
9. Maximize the potential of your profile biographies to make better connections.
10. Measure your research impact online.

Fig. 2.3 How to raise your research visibility [7]

Unique Identifiers

Academics or researchers typically collaborate with colleagues across disciplines and institutions and in other countries. This raises the prospect of interacting with multiple information platforms, each of which may require entry of personal data. Research is increasingly global, and many interactions take place from email to video conferencing and online databases. Researchers have traditionally been identified by their names, but this has never worked reliably because of confusions between popular names, errors in transliteration, and name changes through marriage [8].

If researchers possessed a unique identifier that could ensure that they were credited with all their personal academic research outputs, the academic universe would be much easier. Many consider email addresses, social media accounts or institutional accounts to be unique identifiers. But not all agree on that taxonomy. What is needed is a standard unique identifier. One option is the ORCID Identifier. ORCID is an international, interdisciplinary, open and not for profit organization that has tried to solve the researcher's name ambiguity problem for the benefit of all involved in the research process (see Chap. 4).

ORCID

ORCID® (https://ORCID.org/), Open Researcher and Contributor ID, is an open, non-profit, community-driven effort to create and maintain a registry of unique researcher identifiers and a transparent method of linking research activities and outputs to these identifiers. ORCID is unique in its ability to reach across disciplines, research sectors, and national boundaries. It is a hub that connects researchers and research through the embedding of ORCID identifiers in key workflows, such as research profile maintenance, manuscript submissions, grant applications, and patent applications [4].

It is intended that the ORCID iD number will become the standard unique author identifier in research, much as the digital object identifier or DOI has become for scientific papers and data. The assigned unique identifier will remain associated with the researcher throughout their career. The researcher manages their own record of activities and publications. Activities include presentations, conferences, posters, lectures, and more forms of scholarly works. ORCID has an interface that automates the process of importing new records of publications from PubMed, Scopus, and other major databases.

Many medical journals request authors, either the corresponding author or all authors, to register for an ORCID iD during manuscript submission process and before their papers can be published. The reproducibility and integrity of biomedical science is being heavily scrutinized [6], including the authenticity of authors and authorship, even more so now in the Covid-19 literature [7]. Within that push toward fortifying the integrity of biomedical literature lies the ability to distinguish valid from invalid authors. Given that authorship is central to the integrity of scholarly literature, the editors of many ethics and biomedical journals may be relying on ORCID iDs to screen valid from invalid authors [8].

Research funding agencies are increasingly using ORCID iDs, as reflected by their inclusion in the list of member organizations. As with manuscript submission to journals, the grant application process routinely demands information from applicants, which they have submitted on multiple similar applications in the past. By funding agencies integrating their systems with ORCID it does make the application process easier for researchers. Universities use ORCID identifiers to help them track their own researchers; it is so much easier to automatically compile lists of grants and publications rather than asking for this information from their own staff members [4].

Students in science, medicine, education, STEM, and other research-oriented professions are encouraged to register for an ORCID iDs. ORCID identifiers are very useful for early career researchers who are looking to get funded, published, and to advance their careers. It makes unpublished works more creditable and more visible. The ORCID system also can make certain information private because the profile is self-managed by the researcher.

Which Platforms Do I Use

There are many social media platforms to choose from, so think about the audience you are trying to reach and the impact you want to achieve. You want to identify the best audience to mention attendance at an upcoming conference or promoting a newly published paper. Find out which platforms your colleagues use and focus only on those (see Chap. 8).

For example, on social media platforms, Twitter, or X, is a good platform to share news and information with other academics and the public. Facebook is more of a place where groups with shared interest build community spaces for long-term contact on a specific topic. LinkedIn offers similar spaces but is more focused on connecting professionals in your field, alumni, and other members of your professional organizations. Remember each platform has its own membership characteristics and you have limited time, so try to focus on where to develop a digital profile for your work.

Many researchers create profiles on different Academic Social Networking Sites or ASNS sites. How those sites are chosen by the researchers may be decided if the individual is looking to self-promote or to promote their research and their academic reputation. Having profiles on ResearcherID (Thomson Reuters), Scopus Author Identifier (Elsevier), Publons (Clarivate), Google Scholar, ScienceOpen, arXiv, ResearchGate, Academia.edu, Mendeley, Zotero, etc. is not uncommon.

Having multiple digital profiles can be impractical since a digital profile must be updated and kept current to serve its purpose. Don't post for the heck of it so plan ahead. Schedule weekly or monthly social media posts to promote materials that support your research. Knowing the audience that is using a chosen platform is vital, limiting your profiles to just the relevant platforms and keeping the information current are important steps to establishing your digital identity.

Create Profiles on High-Ranking Sites

Since the time you have to maintain your digital identity is limited, it is best to choose and identify the platforms that will give you the most exposure. To promote your research, you need to know your target audience. Which social media platforms do your colleagues use? Which platforms do your collaborators participate in? Does the conference you are presenting at have a hashtag (#) for the meeting? Are you disseminating your research to a specific group such as genetic researchers? If so, which platforms do they use to communicate, Facebook, blogs or Twitter or X? Are you using social media to raise the "impact" of your research for promotion, or do you need it to be cited?

Make Your Web Address Easy to Locate

Most web addresses on a social media platform can be modified to be easier to locate by switching it to a vanity URL. On LinkedIn you can create your public profile URL. Having a custom public profile URL will help colleagues and collaborators identify your unique profile easily and connect with you. Setting up a custom LinkedIn profile URL is easy to do—if your name is somewhat common, you may need to add in your middle initial or an "phd," or "dr." or "cpa" because LinkedIn has more than 650 million users, many of whom have already set theirs up. This is how your customized LinkedIn profile URL will look: http://www.linkedin.com/in/yourname

Check each platform to see if your "digital profile" has a personalized URL available. Facebook allows for "vanity URL's" that meet certain criteria. A branded Facebook username gives your page an easy to find and easy to share URL that looks professional and branded.

Create a Single Home for Your Online Presence

Setting up your own website or blog is an easy way to manage your digital identity. Many universities offer a digital space for researchers. This is a good space to share research ideas, teaching materials, opinions, and more.

When designing a personal web page think of your landing page as a personal repository for your academic identity; a comprehensive portfolio of your work; a virtual space where you can be in control of aesthetic, content, and structural choices (see Chap. 7).

Your personal website could include resources such as:

- Your CV (either in an interactive form, as a PDF, or both).
- Portfolios of your publications, digital projects, and course websites/syllabi.
- Your teaching statement and/or your faculty diversity statement.
- Links to your publications and other research.
- Links to your social media profiles and ORCiD profile.
- A professional contact page.
- A blog and/or podcast.

Be sure to check with your organization if there are any policies about what content can be shared in this space. If you feel it is too confining, set up a web site that may cost you an annual fee but the web address could be personalized and easier to locate. This could be with a web hosting company such as WordPress, Square Space, Web.com, Wix, or others. That way if you leave an organization, you will still have access to the personalized web site.

Link Your Online Profiles Together

Once you have started to get involved in research, collaborations and have created a few social media accounts, you need to think about linking your professional profiles together. At this point you want to be sure your personal profile accounts are separated from your professional profiles. Be sure the tone of your content is consistent and remains a reflection of your work and not you personally.

ORCID allows "trusted organizations" to link to and update your ORCID profile. This can only be done by the owner of the profile granting permission. Allowing trusted organizations to add information to your record ensures the data connected with your ORCID profile is authoritative and trustworthy, as well as saving you time entering information manually. The organization which added the work to your record will be listed as the source of the item [3]. Some of the trusted organizations include, Scopus Author ID, ResearcherID (Thompsons Web of Science), Open Aire, Europe PubMed Central, HAL (the French multidisciplinary open archive), Japan Link Center (JaLC), Data Cite, and more. A complete list can be found on the ORCID web site.

In an academic world in which decisions on promotion, tenure, and funding often depend on the researcher's scientific impact, an incorrect publication or citation record in an online database can be an impediment. Linking all your profiles together with an ORCID profile is a useful tool.

Write Posts on Other Blogs to Gain Visibility

Authoring a blog post on an established blog can be another way to get your name out there. You can use this post as an opportunity to link to your preferred online profile, your ORCiD profile or your personal website. Many professional organizations or societies have blogs that are hosted on the home page of or linked off the web site. Search for colleagues' blogs, research collaborators or education portals that are always looking for guest bloggers. Many institutions or universities have blogs that are used to promote the careers of their faculty or students.

It is not uncommon for employers, future employers, or potential collaborators to look people up online. Be sure the writing tone of your blog posts are professional and do not include anything you would not want to be quoted on. Everything on social media is public and your digital footprint follows you for life.

Decide If You Will Have a Personal or a Professional Digital Presence

One of the main issues that should be considered, before establishing a digital presence, should be how you will choose to use your profile. Will you combine your professional and personal accounts, or will there be two separate profiles? If you plan to use your social media and other online profiles to spread and influence the impact of your research, you may want to maintain a clear divide between your personal and professional footprints.

In 2021, the American Medical Association (AMA) produced a document on Medical Ethics Professionalism in the Use of Social Media 2.3.2 which states:

> To maintain appropriate professional boundaries physicians should consider separating personal and professional content online [9].

One way to do this is to use different formats of your name, for example "Peggy Dreker" for my personal account, with a personal email address and "Margaret Rush Dreker, MPA, MLS" with a work email address for your professional identity.

Privacy Settings

Whatever the choice of names on your profile, be sure you are aware of all the privacy settings available on each of your account's platforms. Privacy settings will limit what materials are available to the public. Even an ORCID profile allows you, as the administrator of the profile, to restrict information from public view. Every platform has different settings which you should familiarize yourself with.

Researchers tend to be cautious of discussing their papers, sharing data, and making comments on social platforms, whether to protect new discoveries or personal privacy. Therefore, they often prefer to use their own communication channels instead of more public networking platforms [6].

Use Appropriate Images Online

Before you decide to take the leap into using social media platforms, it is suggested that you search your name in a search engine to see what is online about you. You also need to see what images are associated with your name. Most search engines have a tab that allows you to view just images related to your name search. Do images appear that were taken at a professional conference that you spoke at last year? Are the images from a family reunion or from an event that you would prefer was kept private? If that has occurred, review the privacy settings of the platform, and remove the tags of yourself from other people's photos.

Have a professional headshot taken that can be used for any work that you will do including appearing at a conference, presenting at grand rounds or your in house "About Me" page. Many organizations and universities offer this opportunity to faculty or researchers once a year. If you were to have an interview, you would spend a lot of time ensuring that you look well-dressed, professional, and approachable. It is just as important to portray a similar image on any of your digital profile platforms. In a 2017 article, White suggests that choosing the right image may be critical—people's first impressions from profile photos shape important decisions, such as choices of whom to date, befriend, or employ. White and his team concluded that people make suboptimal choices when selecting their own profile pictures, such that self-perception places important limits on facial first impressions formed by others [10].

Whichever profile photo you choose to use online, load it as a high-quality format and use it consistently across any of your digital profiles. That way you can control how you appear in your digital presence.

Maximize the Potential of Your Profile Biographies to Make Connections

Most platforms used to establish a digital identity provide space for you to submit information about yourself as a short biography. You can add a brief biography to your ORCiD record to provide a narrative description about you and your research career and interests. The biography field is a plain-text field limited to 5000 characters. As with all fields in the ORCID record, you can set who can see your biography by choosing your preferred visibility [11].

Since every platform limits the number of characters you can enter in this field be sure to write a short biography that shows your interests, skills, or experiences. Twitter, or X, allows a 160-character biography field. On Twitter, your biography field will appear in the search results when people search for your name. It will be very visible. Twitter is a place to interact with people who are in your field. To be considered part of the group, you must use words that this group relates to and uses.

In LinkedIn your summary is entered in the text box at the top of your LinkedIn Profile; the "About" section. It appears just under your photo. The space that provides 2000 characters where you can give an overview of your professional life. Your summary is the one place you define yourself in your own words. You use it to chart your career, highlight your biggest achievements, or introduce your research interests. The short summary is your chance to personalize and design your first impression to others. Using that same information across all platforms, so it is consistent, can make your digital profile more findable and easier to update.

Disclaimers

It is a growing trend for employers to request employers to add disclaimers to their social media platforms. Disclaimers are important because they inform the reader that one's ideas, comments or thoughts are their own and are not a reflection on the organization of which they are associated with. Common Twitter, or X, disclaimers that are used include:

- Opinions are my own and not the views of my employer.
- My tweets are my own.
- My opinions are my own.
- Tweets are my own and should never be taken seriously.

Disclaimers alone are just words and are not a legal binding document. As you create your online profiles you should still be familiar with your institutional social media policy.

Conclusion

Having a digital profile to clearly identify you as an author and your affiliated research is vital and necessary to the integrity of science. Having a digital identity can also prevent a potential conflict of interest for a researchers' work. The decision to jump into the world of digital and social media platforms is one that should be well planned out before the leap is made. How will I maintain my digital identity? How much time do I have to do so? Do I set these sites up as a university representative or as an individual? Do I know the social media policy of my institution? Do I understand the security settings on each social media account? Do I include pictures on the social media platforms? Which platforms will I use? There are benefits and risks when exploring and establishing a digital identity. Be sure to review them all!

References

1. Luzón M-J. Constructing academic identities online: identity performance in research group blogs written by multilingual scholars. J Engl Acad Purp. 2018;33:24–39. https://doi.org/10.1016/j.jeap.2018.01.004.
2. Jordan K. From social networks to publishing platforms: a review of the history and scholarship of academic social network sites. Front Digit Humanit. 2019;6:5. https://doi.org/10.3389/fdigh.2019.00005.
3. ORCiD: add works to your ORCID record. https://support.orcid.org/hc/en-us/articles/360006973133-Add-works-to-your-ORCID-record. Accessed Jan 2023.
4. Anstey A. How can we be certain who authors really are? Why ORCID is important to the British Journal of Dermatology. Br J Dermatol. 2014;171(4):679–80. https://doi.org/10.1111/bjd.13381.
5. Chaudhary VB. A scientist by any other name. Nat Microbiol. 2022;7(3):351. https://doi.org/10.1038/s41564-022-01067-2.
6. Tran C, Lyon J. Faculty use of author identifiers and researcher networking tools. C&RL. 2017;78 https://doi.org/10.5860/crl.78.2.16580.
7. Kraakevik J. Crafting a positive professional digital profile to augment your practice. Neurol Clin Pract. 2016;6(1):87–93. https://doi.org/10.1212/cpj.0000000000000211.
8. Fenner M, Haak L. Unique identifiers for researchers. In: Bartling S, Friesike S, editors. Opening science. Cham: Springer; 2014. https://doi.org/10.1007/978-3-319-00026-8_21.

9. American Medical Association. Professionalism in the use of social media. https://code-medical-ethics.ama-assn.org/ethics-opinions/professionalism-use-social-media. Accessed Jan 2023.
10. White D, Sutherland CAM, Burton AL. Choosing face: the curse of self in profile image selection. Cogn Res Princ Implic. 2017;2(1):23. https://doi.org/10.1186/s41235-017-0058-3.
11. ORCID: add a biography to your ORCID record. https://support.orcid.org/hc/en-us/articles/360006971513-Add-a-biography-to-your-ORCID-record. Accessed Jan 2023.

Chapter 3
Managing Your Research Identity and the Role of the Librarian

Gerald Shea

Introduction

Libraries, like society, are always changing and the pace of that change increases each year as new technologies continue to impact the profession of librarianship. In this context, the role of academic librarians continues to transform, which makes it essential that academic librarians adapt to the evolving needs and expectations of their users. Furthermore, academic librarians need to be aware of the shifting higher education model and how it impacts our practice.

Universities and, by extension, academic libraries face unprecedented challenges as they enter a new era following the COVID-19 pandemic. Even before the pandemic, the higher education model was under serious pressure from various factors, including an overall decline in student enrollment and decreased state funding for public institutions [1]. One way to help universities, academic libraries, and faculty to thrive in this more challenging environment is to promote the research that faculty are doing at our institutions. Academic librarians are in a good position to assist faculty with scholarly communication; this is crucial for faculty as scholarly impact is one, if not the most important factor, leading to success and promotion. Historically, citations have been the most used method to measure scholarly impact, however citations are only one way to measure research output.

Alternative metrics provide a more multidimensional perspective, e.g., views, shares, and downloads of articles [2]. Academic librarians can help faculty navigate these new, more multifaceted ways to measure the impact of their research. To do this successfully, librarians need to incorporate new digital tools into the work of the profession [3]. As Vassilakaki and Moniarou-Papaconstantinou [4] wrote, "Digital technology and their advanced communication networks have considerably

G. Shea (✉)
Seton Hall University, South Orange, NJ, USA
e-mail: gerard.shea@shu.edu

© The Author(s), under exclusive license to Springer Nature Switzerland AG 2023
M. R. Dreker, K. J. Downey (eds.), *Building Your Academic Research Digital Identity*, https://doi.org/10.1007/978-3-031-50317-7_3

influenced the way research is conducted and research methodologies are adopted by scholars." These technological changes provide the opportunity for librarians to create new research services and to embed these services in scholarly communication initiatives. According to Widen [5] scholarly communication is a broad term used to describe the process of sharing and disseminating a scholar's work first to the academic community and then to the public.

There are three main stages in the scholarly communication process [6]. The first stage is communicating through informal networks by using social media; the second stage is sharing research publicly through conferences and pre-prints; and the final stage is publication of scholarly articles in academic journals. This chapter will discuss the academic librarians' role in helping scholars manage their research identity in the dynamic world of scholarly communication.

At its most basic, the purpose of scholarly communication is for the author to share their research with an audience of readers. Research derives from the middle French word *recerche*, meaning rare [7]. As the derivation of the word suggests, the researcher is engaged in a scholarly process or conversation, meant to create new knowledge. For this conversation to serve its purpose, scholars must be able to effectively share their research.

Researchers may not be familiar with the tools and metrics that are used to both increase scholarly impact and measure it. This provides an opportunity for librarians to use their expertise to assist faculty.

One way that academic librarians might help researchers improve their research identity is through open access publishing, an area faculty are not always familiar with. According to UNESCO [8], open access means "free access to information and unrestricted use of electronic resources for everyone." A commitment to open access (OA) publishing by scholars could lead to wider dissemination of their research findings. Other examples of the evolving model in scholarly communication are the use of social media (see Chap. 8) and alternative metrics (see Chap. 6) by faculty to disseminate and promote their research.

Opportunities to Enhance the Role of Librarians

Librarians are apprehensive to change. However, librarianship has always been expanding and changing. The Hollywood depiction of a library is as a purchaser and repository for collections. Yet, today, we see scholarly communication becoming more recognized as a core competency for the profession. According to Abbott [9], librarianship is a federated profession, meaning librarians are loosely grouped with people doing different kinds of work but sharing a common orientation, and this trait allows for the librarians' role to evolve and be responsive to change. This responsiveness is essential because librarians need to evolve their roles and services to meet changing user needs and expectations [10]. Because of the adaptability of our profession, we should see change as an opportunity to enhance our professional relationships with the teaching faculty and improve the standing of the academic library as an institution. From this point of view, we can see the evolution of scholarly communication as an opportunity for academic librarians and libraries to thrive.

With that in mind, let us look at some of the institutions that are using this opportunity to enhance the role of academic librarians in the scholarly communication process. In this chapter, we will look at three libraries at the University of Houston, University of Minnesota, and Seton Hall University to see what they are doing to embed their librarians in the research activities of their universities.

At the University of Houston, a research services program initiated by the library got turbo charged by a university wide drive to increase research output. At Minnesota, a new university strategic planning initiative provided librarians with the chance to become more integrated in scholarly communication activities. And at Seton Hall, a move from an R3 Carnegie Classification to a high research activity R2 Carnegie Classification afforded librarians with the opportunity to play a bigger role in the research activities of the university.

Starting a Research Services Program

In 2017, librarians at the University of Houston (UH) started a new research services program to support ongoing research at the university. As part of this program, librarians were expected "to understand the changing research process" [3]. As a result of this expectation, job postings for librarians in the program communicated the need for new hires to have experience with or the desire to learn new research technologies.

Clearly, communicating the need for librarians to understand the research process, as the UH program does, is essential, if we, as a profession, would like to play an expanded role in helping faculty manage their research identity. To become more integrated into the research process, we must explicitly state this goal through position postings and in our strategic planning. If we are to be successful, it would also be beneficial to connect our programs to larger university strategic initiatives.

A year after UH Libraries started their research services program, the university launched a drive to increase research output. The program, instituted in 2018 by the president of the university, was called the 50-5 initiative and it encouraged faculty to increase their research output by 50% in 5 years. This commitment by the university to become a more research-intensive institution helped galvanize the UH Libraries' research services program. The urgency created by the 50-5 initiative motivated UH librarians to do more to support the increased research needs of the faculty.

To meet these increased needs, librarians began to meet with faculty collaborators at the university. From these conversations, the research services team determined the biggest need for faculty was helping to cultivate their research identity, i.e., learning how to track and measure their research and its impact. As a result of identifying these needs, "the team learned skills and developed workshops to instruct researchers in how to effectively use researcher profiles, determine their impact using metrics and altmetrics, and determine the best avenues for disseminating their research" [3]. Additionally, subject librarians learned these same skills and conducted outreach to their departments to promote these new services.

As part of their outreach, subject librarians were expected to contribute to the 50-5 initiative by creating opportunities for consultations and collaborations between faculty and the research services team. This kind of cooperation between subject librarians and members of the research services team is crucial if these kinds of programs are to succeed. The subject librarians do not need to be experts in these areas, but they need to be familiar with these tools. The subject librarian along research services can collaborate with each other to best serve faculty of each department [3].

An example of this comes from UH where a faculty member in the College of Technology needed help to disseminate and track the impact of software she had created. In this case, the subject librarian for the College of Technology was able to call on members of the research services team to assist with the request. The subject liaison, the faculty member, and two people from the research services team met to discuss the best tools to help the faculty member track the impact of her software. As a result of this collaboration, the faculty person decided to use GitHub to host her software; GitHub [11] is a platform for software developers to store and collaborate on code and to, "use alternative metrics to track the usage and impact of her software" [3].

Alternative metrics or altmetrics provide information about article citations along with downloads, views, and shares of articles; likes on social media platforms, and retweets on Twitter or X to assess scholarly impact [2]. According to Piwowar [12] these alternative ways to measure the impact of research "give a fuller picture of how research products have influenced conversation, thought and behaviour." She also points out these research products are now more diverse, e.g., data sets, software, and patents.

As the case at the University of Houston shows, the diversity and complexity of both the research products and the tools to measure the impact of that research creates an opportunity for librarians to assist faculty as they attempt to manage their scholarship and scholarly identity. The reality is many faculty members would rather focus on their research and not have to worry too much about how many times they have been shared on social media. This unfamiliarity or even unwillingness of faculty to learn with altmetrics can open the door for librarian intervention.

Changing the Role of Librarians at the University of Minnesota

At the University of Minnesota (UMN), liaison librarians have become more integrated into scholarly communication activities as part of a university wide strategic planning initiative. As part of this strategic change, Karen Williams was recruited to be the first Associate University Librarian for Academic Programs at UMN. The mission for the new division was to make UMN Libraries more central to the academic life of the university by integrating library resources into academic programs. The university aimed to become a top three ranked public research university and this goal opened the door for UMN Libraries to become more involved with scholarly communication [13].

Williams brought a non-hierarchical approach with her from the University of Arizona, which she hoped would make a culture shift easier at UMN Libraries [13]. This shared decision-making ethos paired well with the thinking behind the university's strategic initiative called "Transforming the U" [14]. Williams underlined this by telling Malenfant [13], "upstarts with big ideas are not going to get trampled."

This kind of open-minded approach empowers people to take risks and learn from their mistakes. It recognizes that change is not linear, and we learn through the process of implementation. When administrators give librarians the freedom to try new things, changes around scholarly communication or anything else are more likely to succeed.

Williams wanted to set the appropriate tone for the new division of Academic Programs and in that vein, she thought it was "essential to develop an understanding that we are part of the university and part of higher education" [13]. For librarians, who may sometimes feel like they do not stack up with faculty in terms of research and scholarship, Williams' outlook is a positive corrective. Additionally, she understood from experience that to transform the roles of librarians and to contribute to the "Transforming the U" initiative, it would be imperative to have a clear vision of how that transformation would take place [15].

With that in mind, she intentionally focused on including scholarly communication activities in the work of liaison librarians. She did this by changing the job descriptions of liaison librarians and requiring a performance goal for informing faculty about author rights [13]. This is what was done at the University of Houston where, as noted, position postings included the requirement that librarians would be knowledgeable about the changing nature of the research process. These two examples from the UH and UMN libraries show the importance of clearly communicating expectations when job roles are being reworked.

Including these new job duties in position descriptions at UMN enabled liaison librarians to integrate scholarly communication into their work. To help in this process, a new framework was introduced to make position postings more consistent throughout the libraries. The framework included responsibilities for educating faculty about scholarly communication issues, e.g., helping faculty understand their rights as authors. Some additional responsibilities were contributing to copyright websites, advocating for sustainable models of scholarly communication, working with faculty to understand the changing patterns of scholarly communication, and helping to develop tools to facilitate scholarly communication [13].

In addition to reworking job descriptions, Williams established the Scholarly Communication Collaborative to support librarians with the process of updating their roles. According to Williams, the two main focuses of the Scholarly Communication Collaborative were to "develop and implement as appropriate a coordinated plan for the University Libraries to inform and educate its staff; and recommend appropriate approaches for engaging the campus community in the policy and practical issues that surround the process of scholarly communication" [13].

The Scholarly Communication Collaborative supported liaisons by providing workshops on scholarly communication to educate librarians. They also developed resources for the liaisons, including a presentation on author rights and talking points around issues related to scholarly communication. Guidance like this is invaluable when people and organizations are taking part in a transformative process, especially when some involved with that change may not be completely comfortable with it.

One of the librarians from the UMN Libraries shared her experiences working to inform faculty members in her liaison departments about author rights. She observed, "In every department there's a different hook, a different key." She elaborated more, saying it is necessary to give concrete examples from their journals and societies, "and point out prohibitive language in agreements they actually would be signing" [13].

Librarians working with faculty must be able to understand their context and relate to them on those terms to be credible partners. Another way to work well with faculty is to find the faculty members who edit for journals and serve on disciplinary committees. This may help librarians build stronger relationships with faculty and a bigger role in the scholarly communication system.

An important take away from the UNM case is when people are asked to change their role, they often interpret that change as more work. As a result, librarians at UMN were expected to reduce their workload in other areas such as the reference desk and collection development [13].

It is important to remember that time and resources are finite, so if we decide to prioritize in one area, we need to readjust in other areas. It should also be acknowledged that redefining roles can be controversial and painful. Change makers need to be aware of this and they should not try to force change. Instead, they should start a dialogue and be sensitive to the concerns of their colleagues.

At UMN, Williams started the conversation to get people to think in a new way about library services. She also made it clear that decisions did not need to be made immediately. It was an iterative process where the conversation continued without Williams and then people would come back to her with issues, and she would discuss those issues with them. She saw her role as planting a seed to get the process moving [13].

Scholarly Metrics Reports at Seton Hall University

At Seton Hall University (SHU), librarians have been proactive about engaging and supporting faculty with their research identity. The research services team at University Libraries created a Scholarly Impact Metrics research guide for this purpose [16]. The guide covers why scholarly impact is important and defines many of the different impact metrics that might be used to measure scholarly impact. It also provides guidance for faculty about creating author profiles on different platforms such as Google Scholar.

Librarians at the Interprofessional Health Sciences (IHS) campus have created an author profile checklist to help faculty decide where to set up profiles. The options for faculty profiles include ORCID, Google Scholar, and Scopus.

The benefit of setting up a profile with ORCID is it provides a persistent digital identifier (an ORCiD) that the researcher owns and manages. This identifier is unique, allowing the researcher to be differentiated from other researchers. The researcher can also connect the ORCiD with personal information such as affiliations, grants, publications, and peer reviewed scholarship [17].

Scopus is an abstract and citation database with enriched data and linked scholarly research across a variety of disciplines [18, 19]. Scopus can help researchers enhance their visibility because it fosters the "discovery of research and enables researchers to claim their work, ensuring proper accreditation and supporting career development" [19]. Scopus allows researchers to track their own citations and the citations of other researchers, especially in the hard sciences where it provides excellent coverage. Using Scopus, you can find author profiles, citations per article, total citations, and journal rankings [20].

Additionally, librarians at the Seton Hall Walsh Library and Interprofessional Health Science (IHS) Library provide consultations and workshops covering topics related to scholarly communication and research identity. The workshops provided by University Libraries cover topics such as how to set up an ORCiD, how to use Scopus, and how to get published. There are also workshops on the Inter-University Consortium for Political and Social Research (ICPSR), of which Seton Hall is a member.

ICPSR is an international consortium of approximately 780 academic institutions and research organizations in over 40 countries which provides "training in data access, curation, and methods of analysis for the social sciences research community" [21]. In addition, ICPSR maintains a data archive of more than 250,000 research files in the social sciences. ICPSR is a good option for researchers who would like to share their data. ICPSR also allows researchers to track the use and impact of their research by assisting with obtaining DOIs and citations. It also reviews and improves data submitted by researchers [22].

Seton Hall University Libraries creates scholarly metrics reports to assist faculty with the tenure and promotion process (see Fig. 3.1). These reports include journal rankings, acceptance rates, citations, and statistics from the SHU eRepository, including social media likes and mainstream media mentions. Including information on measures such as acceptance rates can enhance a researcher's identity, especially when their articles are published in competitive journals with low acceptance rates. This kind of information can help with the tenure process, as reviewers from different disciplines are often looking for this type of context and may not be familiar with journals outside their discipline.

Faculty Scholarly Metrics Report Request

University Libraries is looking forward to creating your Scholarly Metrics Report.

If you do not have a profile in SHU's eRepository, we will setup a profile for you. We ask you to send a current cv or links to your where your scholarship lives (personal website or blog, Academia.edu, ResearchGate or discipline specific repositories) to erepository@shu.edu.

Please also forward pre-print copies of your publications. We will check journal copyright policies, but in many cases pre-print articles can be posted. If there is an embargo, pre-prints can often be posted two years after publication. More article attachments in your eRepository profile will help increase your download statistics and viewership in our eRepository.

We also recommend you setup a Google Scholar profile if you do not have one.

Please answer a few questions to help us learn more about your scholarship.

Begin

Fig. 3.1 Seton Hall University Libraries faculty scholarly metrics report request

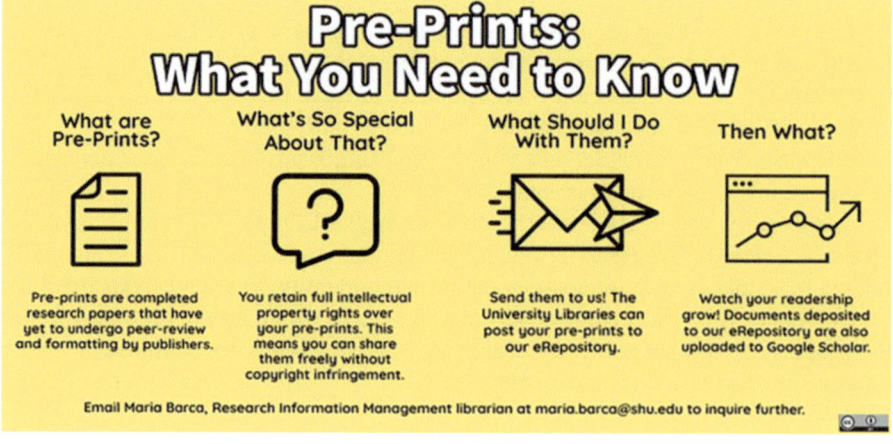

Fig. 3.2 Pre-print information

SHU Librarians recommend to faculty that they create a profile in the SHU eRepository. They also encourage faculty to provide as many of their pre-print publications as possible. A pre-print is the full draft of a research paper in its original form before it is peer reviewed and revised for publication in an academic journal (see Fig. 3.2).

The reason for this recommendation is pre-prints can be shared publicly before the article has been peer reviewed and this increases the visibility of the author's research. Additionally, because the pre-prints are stored in the SHU eRepository, there is no paywall, which also increases the visibility of the research.

Librarians also help researchers contextualize their scholarly contributions by giving them examples of both traditional and non-traditional metrics. Researchers can then begin to collect the relevant information and use it to shape their research identity. Some examples of traditional metrics include citation numbers, journal rankings, and journal impact factors. Examples of non-traditional metrics include news coverage, social media coverage, and ticket sales for faculty in the performing arts.

Librarians also suggest PlumX metrics which can be pulled from the SHU eRepository. PlumX puts metrics into five categories: citations, usage, captures, mentions, and social media. The citation category includes patent citations and clinical citations; the usage category includes non-traditional metrics like clicks and video plays; the captures category indicates that someone would like to come back to the item and includes bookmarks and favorites; the mentions category looks at blog posts, comments on websites, and Wikipedia references; the social media category includes retweets and Facebook likes [23].

Another suggestion SHU librarians give to help faculty provide context and clarity about their research is to explain about name placement in articles they write with multiple authors. For example, the first author is usually the lead author, and it is an important position because it increases the visibility of an author as referencing guidelines mean that readers will see the first author's name, and only et al. will refer to the rest of the authors. However, it is important to note, in some disciplines, the last author position is reserved for the principal investigator. Authors are usually listed according to their relative contribution to the publication. Because there are no uniform rules across disciplines regarding author order, it is important for researchers to clarify the rules that apply to their disciplines.

For scholars who are in disciplines such as Journalism where some of their work is likely to appear in popular publications, e.g., *The New York Times*, which does not provide traditional scholarly metrics. These authors can use circulation statistics and social media metrics show the influence of their scholarship.

Additionally, for researchers who receive grants, it is crucial that they describe the grants they have applied for and successfully earned. The researcher should then explain how these grants advance their research agenda and further how they enhance departmental and university prestige.

Open Access Publishing

Open access (OA) publishing is an option that may enable researchers to have a greater impact. In theory, publishing in an OA journal should result in more access and readership for a research article because of the absence of a paywall [24, 25]. Additionally, most researchers do not realize that publishers allow authors to self-archive pre-print versions of their articles, defined in the previous section, in personal or institutional repositories before publication [25].

There is a good chance scholars will see an increase in their citation numbers if they share their articles by self-archiving. For example, in Physics, authors who made their articles OA by self-archiving saw an increase of between 2.5 and 5.8 more citations [26]. To further this point, a 2014 study of more than 1500 frequently cited European scientists found that these researchers systematically link their publications to self-archived articles on their personal websites or in institutional repositories [27].

According to the Berlin Declaration [28], the goal of OA publishing is to make information "widely and readily available to society." Researchers committed to the OA movement help to make human knowledge and cultural heritage freely accessible to the world. Participating in this movement not only helps society at large, but it also complements the standing of the scholars who contribute to it.

Conclusion

Academic librarians can enhance the scholarly presence of the faculty and universities they serve by sharing their expertise in areas such as author rights, self-archiving, and alternative metrics. By increasing awareness of these issues, librarians will be pushing the conversation around scholarly communication forward in a positive direction. There may be resistance from both faculty and other librarians who are concerned about change, however, it is important to recognize the legitimate concerns of colleagues and not to force change, but to convince people based on the advantages of adopting these new methods and ideas.

References

1. Number of people enrolled in college in the United States from 2017–2022. https://www.statista.com/statistics/1364721/fall-enrollment-us/. Accessed 3 Feb 2023.
2. Bai X, Liu H, Ning Z, Kong X, Xia F, Zhang F, et al. An overview on evaluating and predicting scholarly article impact. Information (Switzerland). 2017;8(3):73. https://doi.org/10.3390/info8030073.
3. Malone A. From liaison to coordinator: how digital humanities influenced a role change and restructure. In: Diamond T, editor. The academic librarian in the digital age: essays on changing roles and responsibilities. Jefferson: McFarland; 2020. p. 84–93.
4. Vassilakaki E, Moniarou-Papaconstantinou V. A systematic literature review informing library and information professionals' emerging roles. New Libr World. 2015;116:37–66. https://doi.org/10.1108/NLW-05-2014-0060.
5. Widén G. New modes of scholarly communication: Implications of Web 2.0 in the context of research dissemination. Amsterdam: Elsevier; 2010.
6. Graham TW. Scholarly communication. Serials. 2000;13(1):3–11.
7. Oxford English Dictionary. Entry: research, n.1. Oxford University Press.
8. UNESCO: what is open access. https://en.unesco.org/open-access/what-open-access. Accessed Feb 2023.
9. Abbott A. Professionalism and the future of librarianship. Libr Trends. 1998;46(3):430.
10. Alvite L, Barrionuevo L. Libraries for users: services in academic libraries. Amsterdam: Elsevier; 2010.
11. GitHub: GitHub's products. https://docs.github.com/en/get-started/learning-about-github/githubs-products. Accessed 25 Feb 2023.
12. Piwowar H. Altmetrics: value all research products. Nature. 2013;493(7431):159. https://doi.org/10.1038/493159a.

13. Malenfant KJ. Leading change in the system of scholarly communication: a case study of engaging liaison librarians for outreach to faculty. Coll Res Libr. 2010;71(1):63–76. https://doi.org/10.5860/crl.71.1.63.
14. Bruininks R. Transforming the U: progress and impact. Rochester: University of Minnesota; 2011. https://hdl.handle.net/11299/108355.
15. Brewer JM, Hook SJ, Simmons-Welburn J, Williams K. Libraries dealing with the future now. ARL Bimonthly Rep. 2004;234:1–9.
16. DeLuca L. Scholarly impact measures. 2023. https://library.shu.edu/facultymetrics. Accessed 21 Feb 2023.
17. ORCID: about ORCID. https://info.orcid.org/what-is-orcid/. Accessed 25 Feb 2023.
18. Elsevier: Scopus: expertly curated abstract and citation database. https://www.elsevier.com/solutions/scopus. Accessed 25 Feb 2023.
19. Elsevier: discover why the world's leading researchers and organizations choose Scopus. https://www.elsevier.com/solutions/scopus/why-choose-scopus. Accessed 27 Feb 2023.
20. For faculty: request scholarly metrics report. https://library.shu.edu/facultymetrics. Accessed 27 Feb 2023.
21. ICPSR: about ICPSR. https://www.icpsr.umich.edu/web/pages/about/. Accessed 26 Feb 2023.
22. ICPSR: start depositing data with ICPSR: who, why, what, and how much is it? https://www.icpsr.umich.edu/web/pages/deposit/index.html. Accessed 25 Feb 2023.
23. Plum analytics: about plum metrics. https://plumanalytics.com/learn/about-metrics/. Accessed 28 Feb 2023.
24. Vadhera AS, Lee JS, Veloso IL, Khan ZA, Trasolini NA, Gursoy S, et al. Open access articles garner increased social media attention and citation rates compared with subscription access research articles: an altmetrics-based analysis. Am J Sports Med. 2022;50(13):3690–7.
25. Ciriminna R, Scurria A, Gangadhar S, Chandha S, Pagliaro M. Reaping the benefits of open science in scholarly communication. Heliyon. 2021;7(12):e08638. https://doi.org/10.1016/j.heliyon.2021.e08638.
26. Harnad S, Brody T. Comparing the impact of Open Access (OA) vs. non-OA articles in the same journals. D-Lib Mag. 2004;10(6) https://doi.org/10.1045/june2004-harnad.
27. Más-Bleda A, Aguillo IF, Thelwall M, Kousha K. Successful researchers publicizing research online: an outlink analysis of European highly cited scientists' personal websites. J Doc. 2014;70(1):148–72. https://doi.org/10.1108/JD-12-2012-0156.
28. Berlin Declaration on open access to knowledge in the science and humanities. 2003. http://www.berlin9.org/about/declaration/. Accessed 27 Feb 2023.

Chapter 4
Managing Your Digital Research Identity with ORCID

Yingting Zhang

Introduction

In the digital era, engaging activities on the internet is a part of daily life. When navigating and working in a virtual space, users inevitably leave their digital footprints wherever they visited, viewed, or interacted. The traces that they left on the internet contribute to their digital representation and reputation, or rather "digital identity." This involves "both the collection of traces (writings, audio/video content, forum messages, sign-in details, etc.) that we leave behind us, consciously or unconsciously, as we browse the network, and the reflection of this mass of traces as it appears after being 'remixed' by search engines." [1].

Digital identity is common and important not only among the general public, but also in the research community. Researchers are using various online platforms to engage in scholarly activities, share research outputs, collaborate with others in their discipline, convey scholarly communications, and build reputations in the research environment. An online presence and digital reputation represent an author's digital identity which often includes their profile, research interests, publications, and professional affiliations among other information in an online platform.

As the number of publications has rapidly increased, researchers strive to make their publications and other types of scholarly works more visible. This visibility allows for quicker and wider attention to their publications in the hope of increasing their research impact. To achieve this goal, it is important for them to cultivate a professional and reputable research identity in the digital environment. A strong digital identity can help researchers and scholars increase their visibility and

---

Y. Zhang (✉)
Robert Wood Johnson Library of the Health Sciences, Rutgers,
The State University of New Jersey, New Brunswick, USA
e-mail: yzhang@rutgers.edu

© The Author(s), under exclusive license to Springer Nature Switzerland AG 2023
M. R. Dreker, K. J. Downey (eds.), *Building Your Academic Research Digital Identity*, https://doi.org/10.1007/978-3-031-50317-7_4

reputation as an expert in their field. A strong digital identity also enables researchers to gauge opportunities to collaborate with others.

Building a strong research identity requires effective management and on-going maintenance. Research identity management is defined as "the practice of scholars and researchers creating and maintaining online identifiers and/or profiles to professionally identify themselves and their scholarly output." [2] There are several ways that researchers can manage their digital identity. Using research networking tools, such as Google Scholar Citations, ResearchGate, or Academia.edu., are common among researchers. Many researchers use these platforms to share their outputs, build a reputation in their specialty, find others' scholarship, and stay connected with their academic community. These platforms, however, do not provide identifiers for the registered researchers.

Some registries and profile systems such as Open Researcher and Contributor ID (ORCID), Scopus Author Profile, and Web of Science Researcher Profiles do provide research identifiers. But they are different in that Scopus and Web of Science are for profit and owned by proprietary companies, while ORCID is a non-profit organization that provides unique persistent digital identifiers to anyone who is interested.

Research institutions and organizations implemented research information management systems (RIMS) or current research information systems (CRIS) to streamline research workflows and to manage grant awards, research data, and faculty publications. The researchers of those institutions can also use RIMS and/or CRIS to track their research, manage collaborations, and share findings.

Some researchers manage their identity via social media, such as LinkedIn or Twitter or X, to post their publications and other scholarly activities. These platforms can be used to retweet information related to their research, and to stay informed of trending topics in their field. Using online repositories (subject specific or generalist) is another way to manage research identities. Researchers use them to distribute their scholarly works widely and promptly. Many academic organizations maintain an institutional repository (IR) for their faculty to deposit publications to comply with their open access policy. By depositing their scholarly works in these repositories, researchers are making their work output more visible, discoverable and accessible, with chances to become more impactful.

A researcher's digital identity, like any other identity, should be safeguarded and protected. Researchers should be cautious and mindful when posting any information on any online platforms. Once it is posted, it leaves footprints that cannot be eliminated. They should also be aware of potential risks to their digital identity such as identity theft or fraud, or damage to reputation. By carefully managing their digital identity, researchers ensure that their online presence is professional, accurate, up to date, and correctly reflective of their interests and accomplishments.

While various systems and ways are available to manage digital identities, this chapter focuses on using ORCID. It describes what ORCID is and its benefits. The chapter will also discuss how ORCID can be used to manage research identities effectively. The chapter also provides guidance for populating ORCID records and connecting ORCID iDs with various research systems and workflows. With the practical information provided in this chapter, readers shall gain a better understanding of how this unique identifier can be used to cultivate their research identity.

What Is ORCID?

ORCID, Open Researcher and Contributor ID, is intended for "connecting research and researchers," as indicated on its website [3]. ORCID is an open-source and non-profit organization established in 2010. Two years later, the ORCID registry was launched. In the registry, researchers can establish an ORCID identifier, known as ORCID iD, which is a 16-digit number, such as 0000-0003-0757-1837. ORCID iD, assigned to any registrant, is a unique and persistent digital identifier that distinguishes a researcher from others, particularly those who bear the same or similar names. The ORCID registry enables researchers to create an ORCID profile free of charge.

Researchers can populate their ORCID record with biographical information, education, employment, funding, and professional affiliations. Scholarly work can be imported from other trusted and reliable sources thanks to the ORCID interoperability structure through its Application Programming Interfaces (APIs). ORCID's APIs integrate ORCID in institutional systems, RIMS, or other resources in the scholarly communication ecosystem to connect faculty and researchers with their research, scholarship, and innovation [4].

ORCID has been increasingly adopted by the research community in the world. As of February 26, 2023, there are 9.29 million records that are considered yearly active records, meaning "those who have either signed into or updated their own records, or used their records to sign into another system in the last 365 days" [5].

ORCID and ORCID iD are sometimes used interchangeably. To avoid confusion and achieve clarity, in this chapter, ORCID is referred to as the organization, while ORCID iD is the identifier. Below is a captured screen illustrating what an ORCID iD and ORCID record look like.{ORCID (Open Researcher and Contributor)} (see Fig. 4.1).

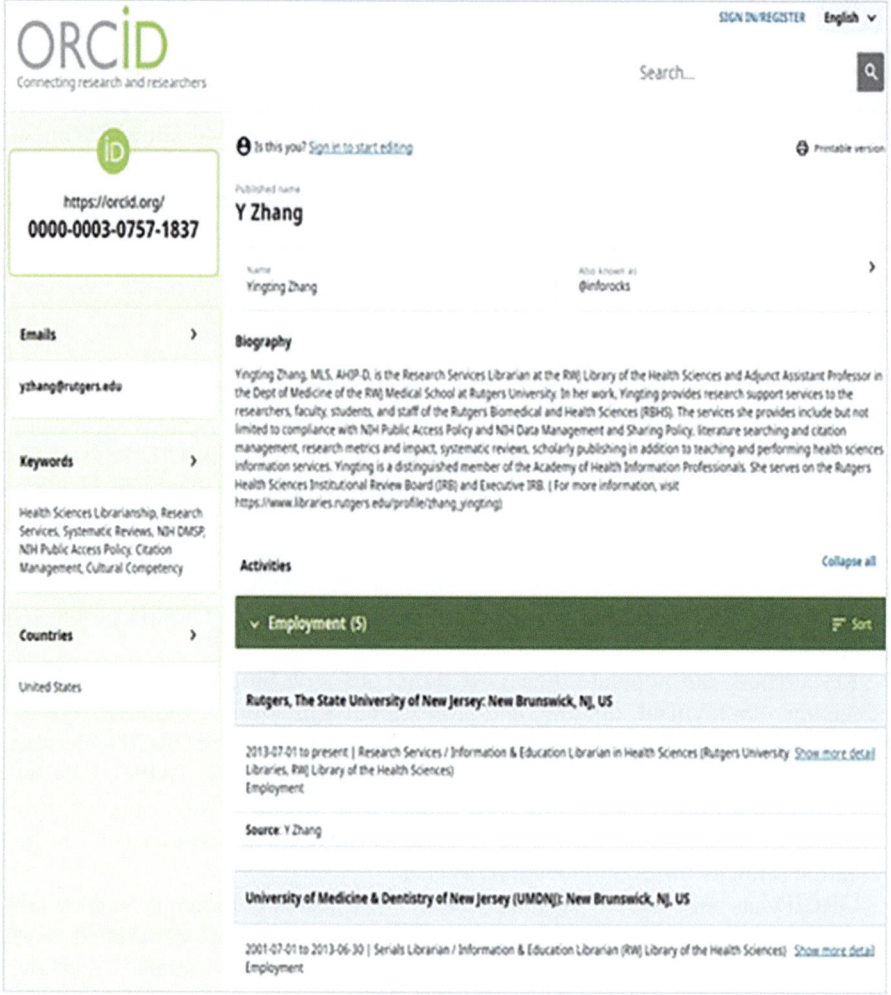

Fig. 4.1 Sample ORCID iD and ORCID record [6]

Benefits of ORCID & ORCID iD

ORCID possesses several characteristics that are beneficial to researchers. ORCID provides a unique and persistent digital identifier that sets one apart from any other researchers through its registry, which is the "core mission of ORCID" as Haak pointed out [7]. Author name ambiguity has long been a problem in the research world. It is usually caused by common, same, or similar names being used by multiple people or by an individual who has used different names (e.g., maiden name, marriage name, translated foreign name, etc.) in his or her scholarship. Name ambiguity causes problems of correct and accurate identification of researchers' outputs

4 Managing Your Digital Research Identity with ORCID

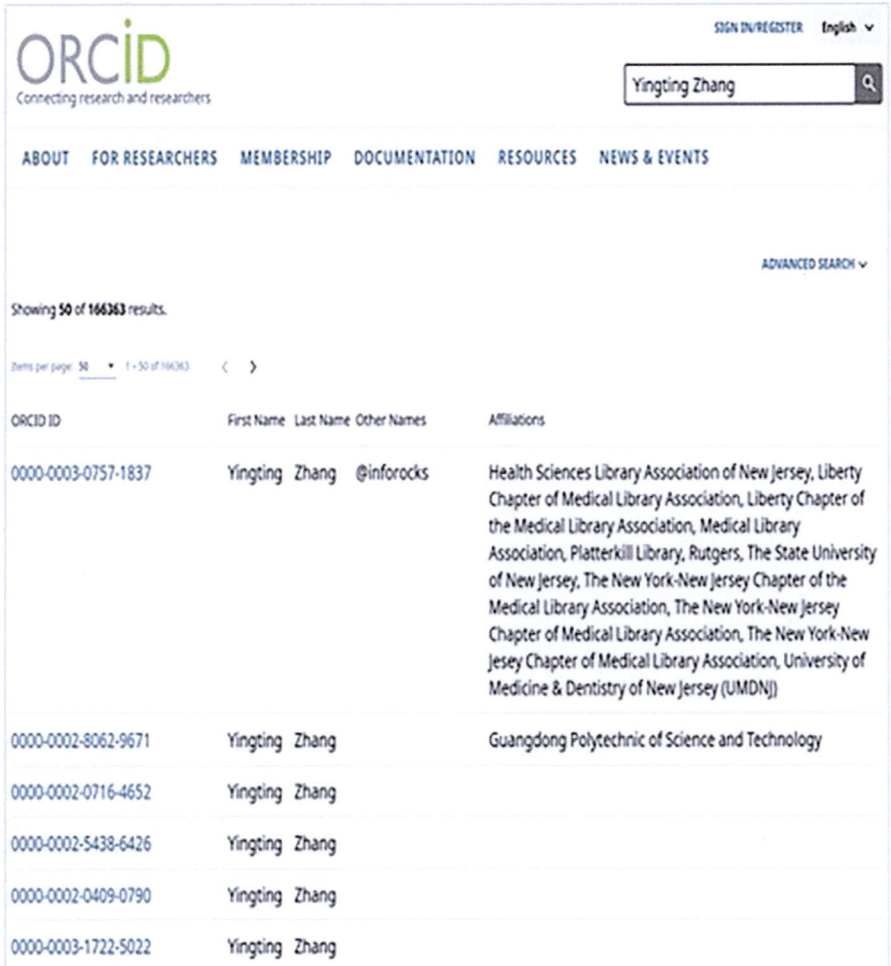

Fig. 4.2 Common Names with Unique ORCID iDs [3]

[8]. The ORCID iD, being unique and persistent, solves the name uncertainty issue. Its uniqueness effectively prevents researchers from being mistaken for other individuals with the same or similar names. For example, the name of this chapter author is quite common when it is spelled out in English (though it is more distinctive in its Chinese characters). Searching Yingting Zhang will retrieve several listings in ORCID. However, each has a unique ORCID iD which differentiates them from one another. Figure 4.2 is an illustration of how ORCID iDs distinguish these records with the same name.

ORCID is free and openly accessible to anyone. Unlike some other digital identifiers issued by proprietary companies with usage restrictions, ORCID can be used by anyone without any conditions. This free access and use of ORCID by individual researchers is made possible thanks to many member organizations and institutions of consortia that paid their institutional membership fees to ORCID [9].

In addition, ORCID is international in scope and has no limitations on geographic areas. Regardless of where it is, anyone in the world who has an internet connection can register in ORCID. Furthermore, is interdisciplinary. It is not specific to certain domains or subject areas. Researchers and scholars of any discipline can use ORCID. Most of the other digital identifiers are discipline or domain specific.

Other benefits of include helping researchers save time by importing or exporting data among various systems. For example, you can add publications from PubMed directly. Using PubMed identifier (PMID) to search from your ORCID record, you can easily retrieve the desired article and place it in your ORCID profile. If there is no PMID, researchers can also add work from a Digital Object Identifier (DOI). A matching record will be retrieved and added to Works Section in the profile.

Scholarly work can also be shared directly from reliable and authenticated resources, such as DataCite, by authorizing any trusted organizations or systems. All this can take place without manually typing the bibliographic information thanks to the interoperability of ORCID's APIs. It makes it possible for researchers to avoid repetitive and tedious manual entry of the same data in each related system, and to achieve data accuracy and efficiency in the research workflows. By fully populating their ORCID records, researchers are able to centralize and showcase all their scholarly works in one authoritative soucce. By integrating their ORCID iDs in other research systems and information resources, researchers make their research and scholarship more visible. This increased visibility allows them to gain more recognition in their field and provides them with more opportunities for research collaboration and scholarly communication. This also ensures they will be fully credited for their scholarly works.

Meeting Stakeholders' Requirements

The ORCID registry is widely supported by the global research community and has been increasingly adopted by various stakeholders such as funders, publishers, institutions, and researchers. Member organizations use the ORCID Member API to facilitate "registration, and information exchange with ORCID records" [10]. With their researchers' permission, the member organizations can use the Member API to add affiliation information, biographical data, funding, peer review, data management plans, and publications to ORCID records.

The connected ORCID iDs help streamline and simplify research workflows. By integrating various online systems including funding agencies' grant applications, reporting systems, publishers' manuscript submission systems, institutional systems, research information management systems, and other types of information systems. Such integrations can help save time and reduce heavy administrative burdens, allowing them to spend more time conducting research. It also makes it easier for stakeholders to view the activities and the overall scholarship of researchers, authors, and contributors. Therefore, more stakeholders are requiring or encouraging the use of ORCID iDs in their workflows and research systems.

Funders are among the adopters of ORCID. For example, Wellcome Trust has required all lead applicants to provide their ORCID iD since 2015 when they complete a grant application in the Wellcome Trust Grant Tracker [11], an online grant application and management system. In July 2019, the National Institute of Health (NIH), the Agency for Healthcare Research and Quality (AHRQ), and the Centers for Disease Control and Prevention (CDC) announced that ORCID iDs would be required for individuals supported by research training, fellowship, research education, and career development awards effective on January 25, 2020 (Notice Number: NOT-OD-19-109) [12].

In April 2020, the U.S. Department of Energy Office of Scientific and Technical Information (DOE OSTI) led to launch the US Government ORCID Consortium, for "bringing together US Government and DOE-affiliated organizations looking to use, adopt, and integrate with ORCID" [13]. All US federal agencies and offices are eligible to join the consortium. The National Security Presidential Memorandum-33 (NSPM-33) issued by the White House in 2021 directs that federal funding agencies to establish policies on requiring individual researchers to use a digital persistent identifier (PDI) in the disclosure of information when applying for grants [14]. The Memorandum defines that 'the term "digital persistent identifier" or "digital persistent identifiers" means a unique digital identifier that permanently and unambiguously identifies a digital object or an individual' [14]. The ORCID iD, being unique, digital, and unambiguous, is ideal to fulfill this federal requirement.

According to Lyrasis, "ORCID is currently the only PID for individuals that meets the requirements stipulated in the NSPM-33 guidance" [15]. It is reasonable to see that it is becoming a norm for funding applicants to include their ORCID iD in submitting grant proposals.

Journals and publishers are also increasingly adopting ORCID which ensures that researchers, authors, and contributors are fully credited for their work. Many journals and publishers are becoming ORCID member organizations. This enables their authors' ORCID iDs to be associated when submitting their manuscript in the journal submission system for publication. For example, PLOS (Public Library of Science) has required all corresponding authors to provide an ORCID iD in their submissions since 2016 [16]. IOP (Institute of Physics) Publishing required all corresponding authors to have an ORCID iD in their ScholarOne account starting September 11, 2017 [17]. ScholarOne Manuscripts is a popular software for article submission, journal workflow management tool, and peer review service used by many publishers and societies [18, 19].

Other contributors such as authors, reviewers, editors, etc. are also encouraged to register for an ORCID iD and use it in their scholarly content. In 2017, Wiley started to require all submitting authors to have an ORCID iD and provide it in the submitting process [20]. When a contributor does not have an ORCID iD, the requiring publishers usually provide an option for them to create an ORCID iD and associate it with the publishers' submission systems.

Many universities and research institutions have participated in consortia to become ORCID member organizations. Rutgers University launched a university-wide implementation of ORCID@Rutgers in 2017 [21]. As of February 1, 2023, 14,129 ORCID iDs were associated with Rutgers domain (rutgers.edu). There were 6582 ORCID iDs integrated with Rutgers system, connected to Rutgers NetIDs, according to the ORCID member portal. Researchers whose Rutgers NetID is connected to their ORCID iD are displayed in the university's public directory. This makes their research and scholarship publicly viewable and allows them to have a single sign-on (SSO) to log into ORCID accounts by using the institutional NetID and password.

By connecting ORCID iDs to the member institutions' systems, both institutions and their affiliated researchers, can enhance individual and institutional research reputation. The number of research institutions becoming ORCID members is increasing. In August 2022, responding to the federal agencies' requirement for use of persistent digital identifiers when applying for grants, the University of Denver is now requiring all its researchers to obtain ORCID iDs and ORCID records [22].

Integrating and Using ORCID iDs in Research Tools and Resources

ORCID iD can be integrated not only with the systems of funders, publishers, universities, and research institutions, but also in research supporting tools, such as Science Experts Network Curriculum Vitae (SciENcv) [23]. SciENcv, a tool for creating biosketches for researchers in application for federal funding, and the DMPTool [24], which is used for developing data management plans in compliance with funders' requirements.

SciENcv is a publicly accessible researcher profile system developed by the National Center for Biotechnology Information (NCBI), a division of the National Library of Medicine (NLM) at National Institute of Health (NIH). SciENcv is available in the My NCBI platform and can be freely accessed via many options, including ORCID. Below is a screenshot (see Fig. 4.3) to show how to sign up for My NCBI with ORCID to use SciENcv.

Researchers who apply for funding from federal agencies like NIH and the National Science Foundation (NSF) must include an appropriate and formatted biographical sketch, or biosketch, in their grant applications and progress reports. A biosketch is intended to highlight a researcher's qualifications and relevant experience for his or her role in a proposed research project. Both NIH and NSF require researchers to submit an appropriate and formatted biosketch in their grant applications or renewal submissions.

Fig. 4.3 Sign up options for SciENcv/NCBI via ORCID [25]

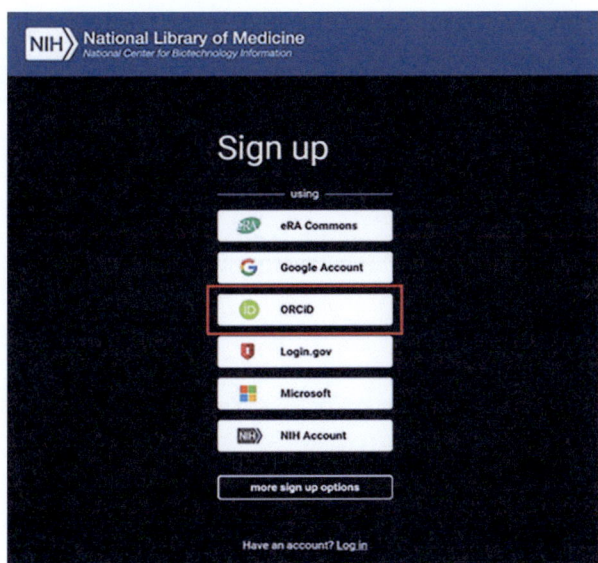

For NIH grants, there are two types of bioksketch format pages. One is the NIH Biosketch and the other is the NIH Fellowship Biosketch format, both required for the senior/key personnel and other significant contributors. NIH Biosketches are limited to five pages. Researchers can use either the Word template or SciENcv to develop a formatted biosketch in applying for or renewing federal grants or submitting research performance progress reports (RPPR). Using a Word template will involve manual work and may exceed the page limit. SciENcv, however, can guide the user to develop the biosketch in the required format within the allowed number of pages. It also leverages data from other systems, such as eRA Commons, My Bibliography, and ORCID. To save time and reduce mistakes, when creating a biosketch, researchers can integrate their ORCID iD in SciENcv, or My NCBI to directly pull the data (biography, education, employment, awards/grants, and scholarly works) from their ORCID record to SciENcv. Figure 4.4 shows using data from ORCID to create an NIH biosketch:

By reusing the data available in ORCID, researchers do not have to reenter their biographic and scholarly data in SciENcv, which can be laborious, tedious, and time consuming. This not only helps them reduce administrative burden but also reduce careless errors.

The DMPTool is an open-source online system that was developed by the California Digital Library. This tool is intended for use by researchers to develop data management and sharing plans, often known as DMPs, as required by many funding agencies including federal agencies and non-governmental funders. The click-through wizard in the DMPTool allows researchers to create a DMP in a format that meets funder requirements. Context sensitive instructional information is also provided to guide the tool users in developing the DMPs. The DMPs developed

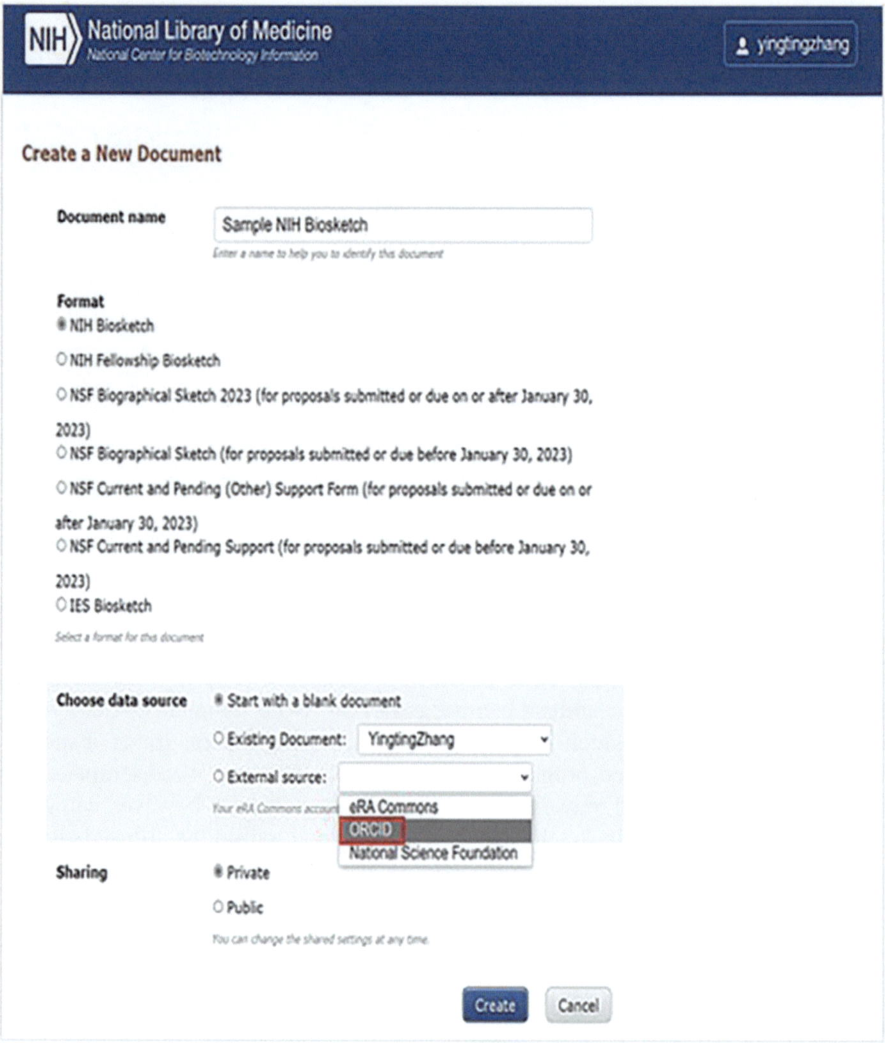

Fig. 4.4 Create a new document using ORCID as a data source [23]

and generated from DMPTool can be included in the grant applications, progress reports, or renewal submissions. They can be made publicly viewable or kept private. The DMPTool can generate DMP IDs which are persistent and unique identifiers for plans created with the tool. By connecting the DMP ID to an ORCID record, researchers authorize the DMPTool to add a DMP to the associated ORCID record. This means the DMP can be automatically pushed from the DMPTool to the Works Section of the connected ORCID record, as ORCID recognizes a DMP as a resource type. The inclusion of DMPs in your scholarly works presents a more complete overview of your research activities.

Populating and Maintaining Your ORCID Record

Creating an ORCID iD is quite easy and simple. However, populating and maintaining your ORCID record is often neglected. Many researchers leave their record blank after they created an ORCID iD during the manuscript submission process or grant application time to meet the requirements of a publisher or a funder. Some may deliberately keep their record content private. While having an empty ORCID record does not make non-incompliant with those requirements, it does disappoint some readers.

Properly populating your ORCID record and keeping it accurate, current, and professional is just as important as registering for an ORCID iD. The ORCID record contains the following sections: Employment, Education and Qualifications, Invited Positions and Distinctions, Membership, and Service. Researchers need to manually add the information by clicking the Add feature on the right side of the section header and filling in the fields of a pop-up window.

For the Funding Section, there are two options to populate the data: by using the Search & Link wizards or adding manually. The section that usually requires the most work and needs to be constantly updated is the Works Section, as researchers conduct research and publish their research findings on an on-going basis.

There are several ways to add Works to an ORCID record which includes using the Search & Link wizards, adding DOI, PMID, adding a BibText file, or adding works manually. Below is an illustration (see Fig. 4.5) of the options for adding works:

It is worth noting that to use the Search & Link wizards, you need to authorize the external systems as trusted parties, so that the systems can interact with each other.

Researchers are often remarkably busy and have little time for administrative work. It is possible for them to assign a trusted individual as a delegate to help populate and/or maintain their ORCID records. The delegation can be set up by clicking the ORCID record name and choosing Trusted Parties. At the bottom of the screen is the section for Trusted Individuals where a researcher can search for an ORCID user to add as a trusted individual. The trusted person must have his or her ORCID record in order to access the researcher's profile. Figure 4.6 shows the section of adding trusted individuals:

As a researcher, you have total control of the visibility of your ORCID record. You decide which part of the record can be viewed publicly and which part is kept private. The settings can be changed when it is needed. What is most important, is to keep the ORCID record accurate, current, and professional, as your digital identity represents who you are as a scholar, what you do and how much you have accomplished in your area of expertise. A well-developed and timely maintained digital research profile will enhance your credibility, visibility, and professional reputation.

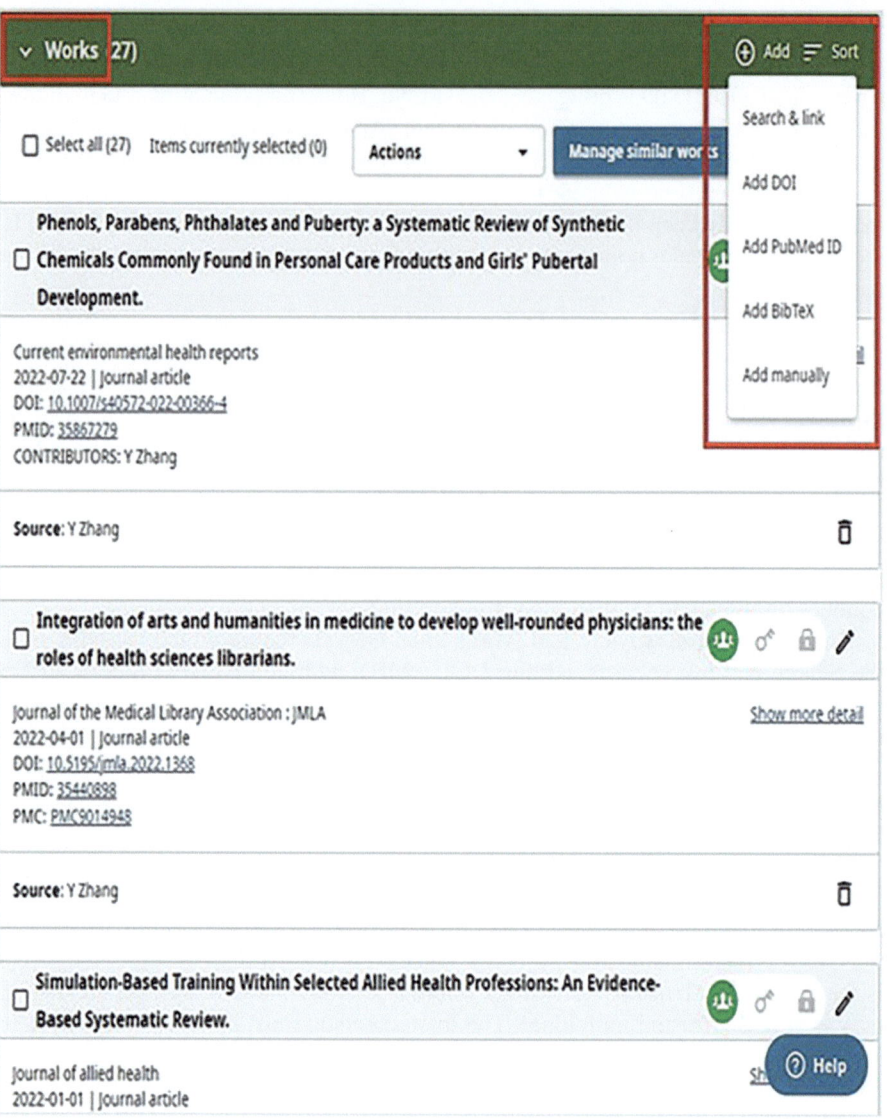

Fig. 4.5 Add scholarly works in an ORCID record [6]

4 Managing Your Digital Research Identity with ORCID

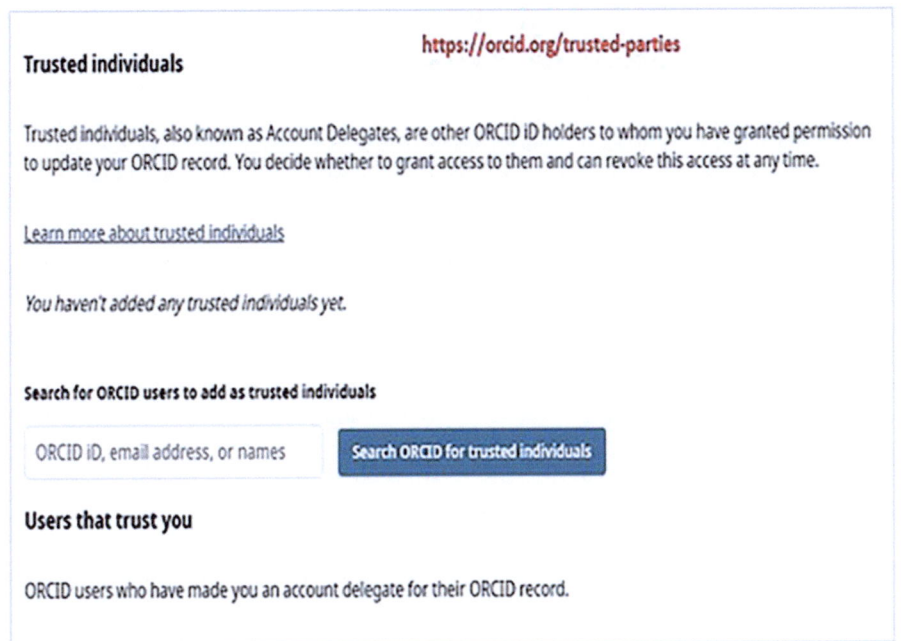

Fig. 4.6 Adding a trusted individual as a delegate [3]

Conclusion

Researchers should cultivate a strong and reputable research digital identity in today's digital world. It makes their research more visible, discoverable, accessible, and recognizable. It also provides researchers with more opportunities to collaborate with others in their field. Researchers should make every effort to manage and to keep their identity professional, accurate, current, and accountable. While there are several ways to manage digital identities, ORCID is being increasingly used to manage and promote professional identities. The fact that it is free and available to all in the world makes it easy to be adopted. An ORCID iD, being a unique identifier to distinguish researchers from any other bearing the same or similar names, solves the ambiguity problem in research. With this function and many additional benefits, ORCID is considered a desirable digital management tool for researchers.

References

1. Ertzscheid O. What is digital identity? Marseille: OpenEdition Press; 2016. http://books.openedition.org/oep/1235.
2. Craft AR. Electronic resources forum - managing researcher identity: tools for researchers and librarians. Ser Rev. 2020;46(1):44–9. https://doi.org/10.1080/00987913.2020.1720897.
3. ORCID. https://orcid.org/. Accessed 18 Jan 2023.
4. ORCID: about ORCID. https://info.orcid.org/what-is-orcid/. Accessed 18 Jan 2023.
5. ORCID: ORCID statistics. 2023. https://info.orcid.org/orcid-statistics/. Accessed 20 Jan 2023.
6. Zhang Y. 0000-0003-0757-1837. https://orcid.org/0000-0003-0757-1837. Accessed 2 Feb 2023.
7. Haak LL, Fenner M, Paglione L, Pentz E, Ratner H. ORCID: a system to uniquely identify researchers. Learn Publish. 2012;25(4):259–64. https://doi.org/10.1087/20120404.
8. Shin D, Kim T, Choi J, Kim J. Author name disambiguation using a graph model with node splitting and merging based on bibliographic information. Scientometrics. 2014;100(1):15–50. https://doi.org/10.1007/s11192-014-1289-4.
9. ORCID: ORCID membership benefits and fees. 2023. https://info.orcid.org/membership/. Accessed 6 Feb 2023.
10. ORCID: member API. https://info.orcid.org/documentation/features/member-api/. Accessed 19 Jan 2023.
11. Wellcome Trust: why does Wellcome support ORCID? https://wellcome.org/grant-funding/open-researcher-and-contributor-id-orcid. Accessed 6 Feb 2023.
12. National Institutes of Health (NIH), US Department of Health and Human Services (DHHS), USA.gov. Requirement for ORCID iDs for Individuals Supported by Research Training, Fellowship, Research Education, and Career Development Awards Beginning in FY 2020. 2019.
13. U.S. Department of Energy Office of Scientific and Technical Information (DOE OSTP): US Government ORCID Consortium. https://www.osti.gov/pids/orcid-services/us-gov-orcid-consortium. Accessed 6 Feb 2023.
14. The White House: Presidential Memorandum on United States Government-Supported Research and Development National Security Policy. 2021. https://trumpwhitehouse.archives.gov/presidential-actions/presidential-memorandum-united-states-government-supported-research-development-national-security-policy/. Accessed 15 Feb 2023.
15. Lyrasis: NSPM-33 & ORCID: information for research organizations. 2022. https://lyrasisnow.org/nspm-33-orcid-information-for-research-organizations/. Accessed 15 Feb 2023.
16. PLOS. Author credit: PLOS & ORCID update. The Official PLOS Blog. 2016. https://theplosblog.plos.org/2016/01/author-credit-plos-orcid-update/. Accessed 15 Feb 2023.
17. IOP Publishing: ORCID. 2017. https://publishingsupport.iopscience.iop.org/orcid/. Accessed 15 Feb 2023.
18. Degele L. Instruction guides available for sites using ScholarOne manuscripts (formerly Manuscript Central). Editors Bull. 2013;8(2–3):60–2. https://doi.org/10.1080/17521742.2012.759773.
19. Clarivate: ScholarOne. 2023. https://clarivate.com/products/scientific-and-academic-research/research-publishing-solutions/scholarone/. Accessed 25 Feb 2023.
20. Citrome L. Open researcher and contributor ID: ORCID now mandatory for Wiley journals. Wiley Online Library. 2016;70:884–5. https://doi.org/10.1111/ijcp.12912.
21. Zhang Y. Librarians promoting and supporting ORCID@Rutgers. Against Grain. 2021;33(4):49–50. https://doi.org/10.7282/00000153.
22. University of Denver: researchers required to obtain ORCID. 2022. https://www.du.edu/news/researchers-required-obtain-orcid. Accessed 15 Feb 2023.

23. National Center for Biotechnology Information (NCBI): SciENcv: Science Experts Network Curriculum Vitae. https://www.ncbi.nlm.nih.gov/sciencv/. Accessed 7 Feb 2023.
24. California Digital Library (CDL): DMPTool. 2023. https://dmptool.org/. Accessed 7 Feb 2023.
25. National Library of Medicine: National Center for Biotechnology Information Sign Up. https://account.ncbi.nlm.nih.gov/signup/?back_url=https%3A%2F%2Fwww.ncbi.nlm.nih.gov%2Fsciencv%2F. Accessed 18 Jan 2023.

Chapter 5
Tools for Managing Your Digital Research Identity

Layal Hneiny

Introduction

As a part of the scholarly world, we know that the research landscape has evolved. Research is a must, not a choice for healthcare practitioners. Research is an essential part of the career promotion process, staying abreast of clinical practices changes, and sometimes integrated into the residency application process [1]. Given that communication and technology are the ingredient of scientific communities [2] and the advent of the internet, it is inevitable nowadays for researchers who are serving on editorial boards, writing papers, peer-reviewing other papers not to strengthen their online presence and visibility, rather to boost their research digital identity and research impact.

This chapter aims to present tools that provide traditional metrics and altmetrics and how these play an important role in a researcher's career. It will look at tools that will increase your online presence to clear up any vagueness with regards to name ambiguities, affiliations and research disciplines.

Free Tools

There are many free tools that help researchers manage their digital research identity such as: institutional repositories," PubMed Profile, Loop, LinkedIn, Doximity, ResearchGate, and others.

The original version of this chapter was revised. The correction to this chapter can be found at https://doi.org/10.1007/978-3-031-50317-7_11

L. Hneiny (✉)
University of South Dakota, Sioux Falls, SD, United States
e-mail: Layal.hneiny@usd.edu

Institutional Repositories

Not only do the institutional repositories, which are freely built websites, allow researchers to archive their outputs, but they also grant them the opportunity to use their outputs. This will increase the number of citations of their work, increasing their visibility and enhancing their scholarly outputs [3] (see Fig. 5.1).

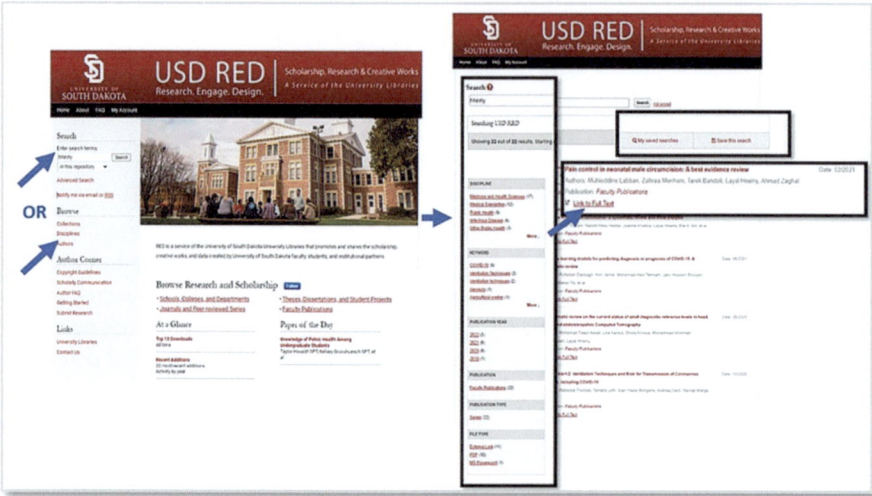

Fig. 5.1 Self-archiving in Institutional Repositories increases probability of citation count and research collaboration. (University of South Dakota Institutional Repository Portal, 2023)

PubMed Profile

My NCBI dashboard preserves researcher's information from saved searches, collections, email alerts, filters, etc. The "My Bibliography" component remain private until the researcher chooses to share the URL. This is one of the tools in the My NCBI dashboard. The citations to the researchers' published journal articles that are indexed by PubMed can be pulled from PubMed, form a file, or added manually into a "My Bibliography" collection to keep the collection dynamic and up to date.

One path for researchers to share their publications into their Curriculum Vitae (CV), website, or blog is via embedding the URL provided by PubMed under "My Bibliography" collection which is one of the many tools in the My NCBI dashboard as outlined in the "My NCBI Help Manual." Another way to embed the URL into a blog or website is by copying the publications in "My Bibliography" collection into a new collection and change the Settings/Sharing of the collection to Public (see Fig. 5.2).

The value of sharing this URL lies in being granted the opportunity to check the full text access of the journal articles through article linkers provided by the institutions. If they are subscribed to certain journals or through PubMed Central or Open Access links, this creates a wider dissemination of one's research, potentially increasing ones citation counts.

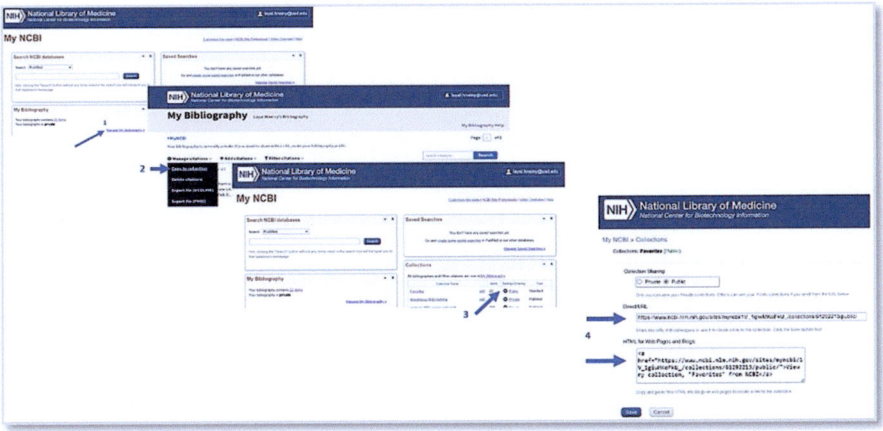

Fig. 5.2 Steps on how to embed researcher's list of publications into other websites

Loop

Loop, created by Frontiers Media SA. and officially launched in 2015, is a universal open science research network for academics that seamlessly maximizes the impact of the researchers and their discoverability of their published work. It connects them with leading academics and colleagues and promotes staying current with new research. The platform provides both the researchers and the public with statistical data such as the number of profile views, publications, researcher views, and the number of the publications downloaded via Frontiers. Upon signing in one can see a more analytical breakdown of the data.

All Frontiers authors have a loop profile (see Fig. 5.3) which is automatically linked to their papers on Frontiers. It provides a CV-like platform, where the public can read the researchers' brief biographies, their current or past affiliation, their education, any honors and awards, as well as organizational memberships. Loop does not only pull articles written by authors in Frontiers but also from many other online resources making it easy for researchers to display their publications (see Fig. 5.4).

Additionally, Loop has worked in conjunction with ORCID (see Chap. 4) to link and synchronize the researcher's profile eliminating the need to maintain multiple online profiles [4].

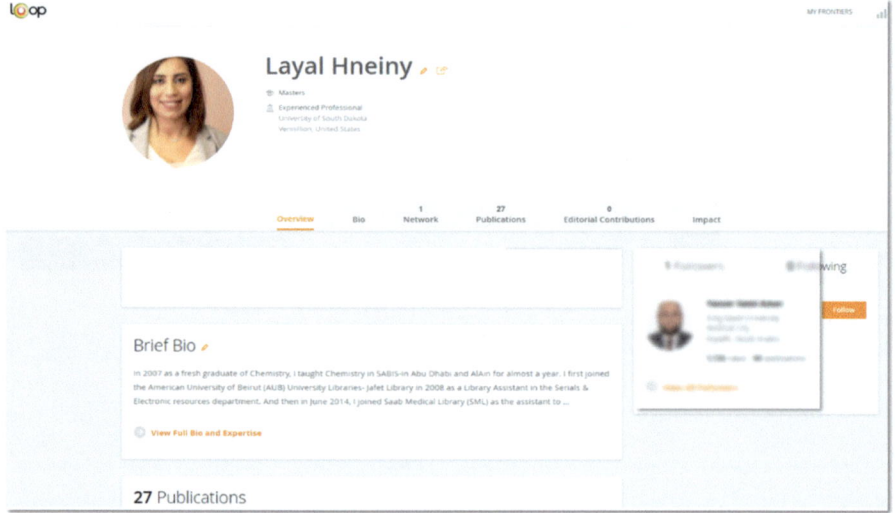

Fig. 5.3 A glimpse into the overview in Loop's platform

5 Tools for Managing Your Digital Research Identity

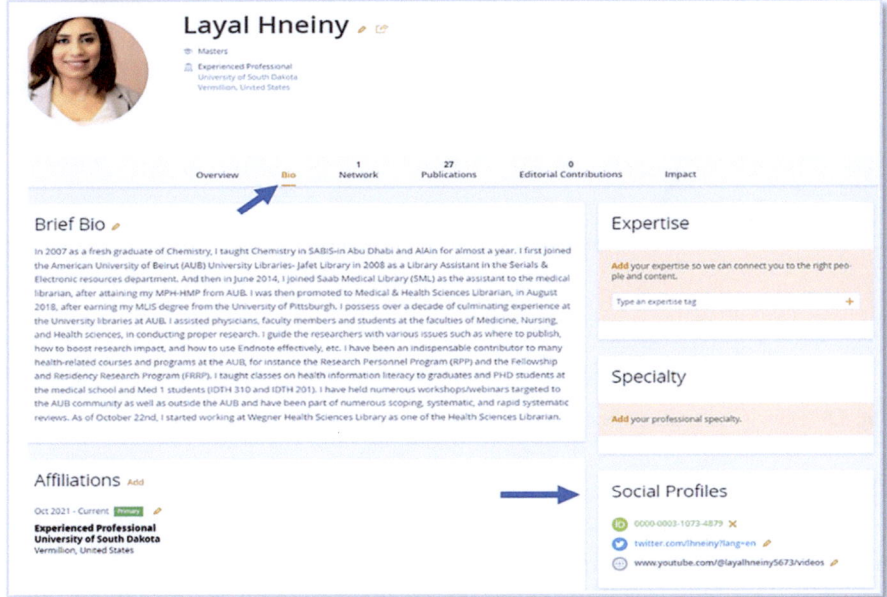

Fig. 5.4 How is ORCID incorporated within loop

LinkedIn

LinkedIn is a business and employment-oriented social and professional media network platform. The LinkedIn platform is an essential tool for any researcher's career. It permits institutions and the research community to extract useful information [5]. This information includes a researcher's field of interest and published work. The LinkedIn platform allows a researcher to freely upload their CV. This includes researcher's experience, education, skill, publications, licenses and certifications, interests, language, courses, and analytics. The user profile is free and visible to the public. It is recommended for any researcher to build a LinkedIn profile.

In addition, a user can easily associate their institutional email address as shown in Fig. 5.5. This can reduce any profile or information ambiguity and maintain consistency.

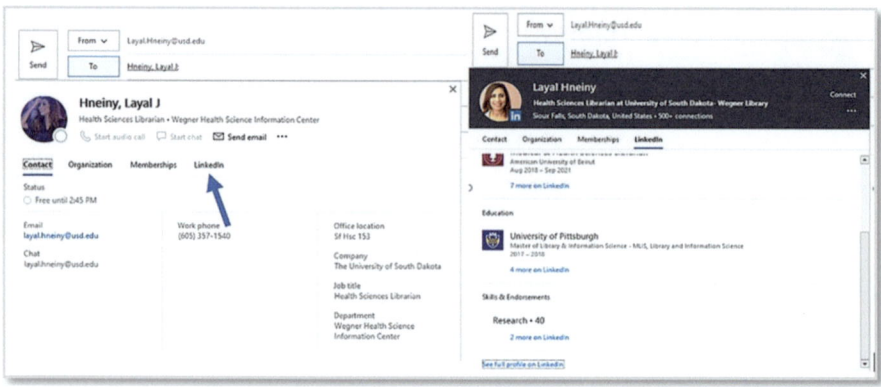

Fig. 5.5 How is LinkedIn embedded in the researcher's institutional email

Doximity

Another tool to establish a researcher's name is to make Doximity profile publicly available. Doximity, www.doximity.com, is another example of a professional medically-tailored network site that consists of a comprehensive database of more than one million US physicians, medical students, and clinically licensed healthcare professionals [6]. As of 2023, approximately 80% of US's physicians and 50% of Nurse Practitioners and Physician Assistants are verified members of Doximity [7].

The importance of having a Doximity profile is that it is searchable and viewable by colleagues. This can open channels to connect with colleagues with similar clinical specialties and interests. Similar to LinkedIn, Doximity is a platform that researchers can seek career opportunities. It allows its members to upload their CVs [8].

Doximity facilitates a transparent look of the training residency programs that are powered by peer nominations, hand-written reviews, and ratings. This allows medical students and physicians to understand and compare the Doximity rankings. According to a study done, with Orthopedic Surgery program rankings, Doximity played a key role in identifying the reputation of the program [9].

It is essential to highlight the synergetic relation between social media visibility and Doximity rankings. It is significant for residency programs to enhance their social media presence [10].

ResearchGate

ResearchGate (RG) is an academic social network site that motivates researchers to embrace the self-archive culture in academia. Share their information in order to increase their self-efficacy, learning, professional growth, accessibility, publicity and reputation. This will boost social media engagement and communities' interests in their topic of research [11].

RG also enables researchers to feature up to five of their research products (including papers, datasets, and chapters) in its "Research" section on their profile page (see Fig. 5.6). By featuring their research, scholars are able to focus on their academic achievements and to contribute to the larger scientific community through dissemination [12].

Like Doximity, there is a presence of RG on social media which presents to researchers the mentions of their work on Twitter or X and Wikipedia and displays them on their profile. This gives a peak on the altmetrics, in addition to the traditional metrics, that RG offers.

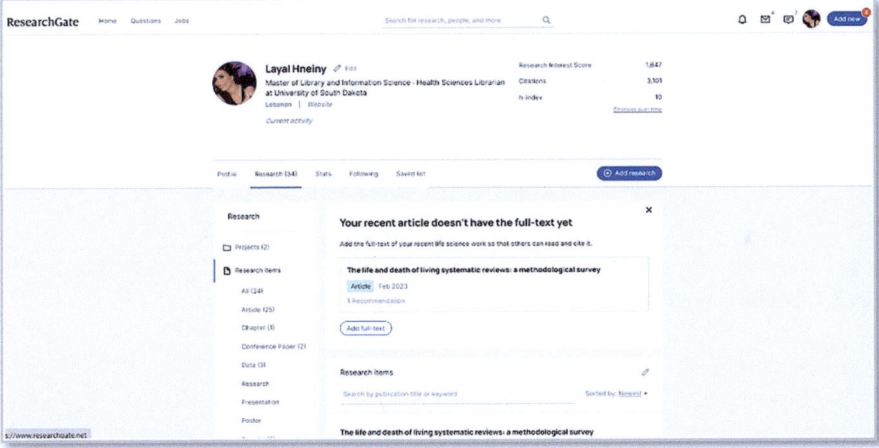

Fig. 5.6 RG platform- Research section

University Webpages

Another way to amplify one's scholarly output is via a university's faculty website. Some universities provide a faculty platform geared to accommodate and advance their e-visibility and self-promotion in a standardized manner across the institution (see Fig. 5.7).

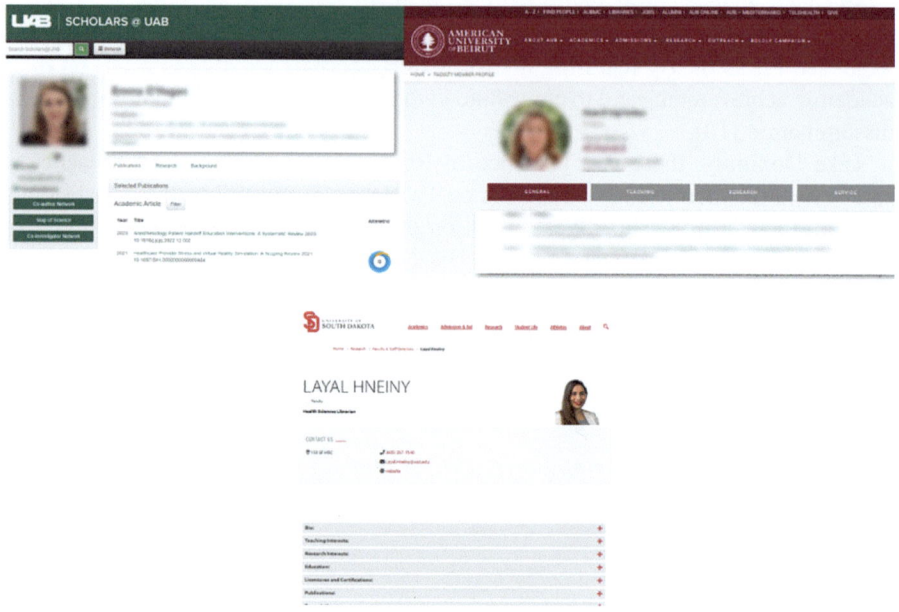

Fig. 5.7 Different profiles of different faculty from different universities

More Tools (see Table 5.1)

Table 5.1 More tools

Source	Website	Description
Academia.edu	www.academic.edu	A platform for sharing academic research, more then 47 million papers have been uploaded and 89 million academic, professional and students read the papers on this platform every month
Wix	www.wix.com	Wix provides powerful technology which allows everyone to get online with a personalized professional web presence with over 200 million users world-wide
Word Press	www.wordpress.com	A free open-source content management system written in hypertext, pre-processed language. Allows you to host website or blog providing personal domain names with 409 million unique visitors per month and over 70 million new posts per month

Bibliographic Analysis Tools

Before introducing "alternative metrics" or Altmetrics analysis, it is important to understand traditional metric analysis., Bibliometric analysis is the analysis of scientific research publications using statistical methods yielding many bibliometric indices intended to measure the individual researcher's output [13]. The Hirsch index (h-index) does not account for the number of years the researcher started his/her career. It does not consider the higher numbers of citations in any publication(s), yet it is still used by most of the academic community.

The h-index is considered a robust and reliable indicator of scholarly achievement because it evaluates the cumulative scholarly impact of researcher's performance by accounting for productivity and citations. In other words, it calculates both the quantity and the quality of the researcher's work in a whole number which reflects neither few papers highly cited nor too many papers with very few citations [14]. The h-index requires access to an author's entire bibliography and citation history. There are platforms that are subscription-based such as Scopus-Author ID and Web of Science (WoS)-ResearcherID, or Google Scholar (GS) Profile which are available to the researcher that are able to calculate and show this number [15].

The calculated h-index in each of the platforms may vary depending on the number of publications and the number of citations reported for the researcher on each platform. Additionally, the presence of authors with identical names can distort the calculation of the h-index making it inaccurate [15]. The feature in Scopus and WoS eliminates the issue of duplication and correct author identification.

Scopus Author ID

Scopus (Elsevier) allows an individual to search and find documents written by a particular author, even if the author's name might be listed inconsistently. Each author is provided a different Scopus Author Identifier (Author ID) which is a numerical value automatically generated by Scopus. Each author profile provides the data which includes the researchers h-index, citation, and publication counts. Multiple entries of the same author can be misleading and yields incomplete bibliometrics. The Scopus database addresses the issue of author's name variation used throughout his/her career and allows the reconciling of multiple entries into a one more comprehensive profile.

In addition to the h-index and other citation information, the profile displays the various names used over the researcher's career, co-authors, and awarded grants (see Fig. 5.8). These fields can increase the opportunity for new collaborations. Researchers should link their author's Scopus profile number into their CVs, blogs, or websites. Scopus is ORCID compliant, and Scopus Author ID can be embeddedinto a ORCID profile allowing more visibility (see Fig. 5.9).

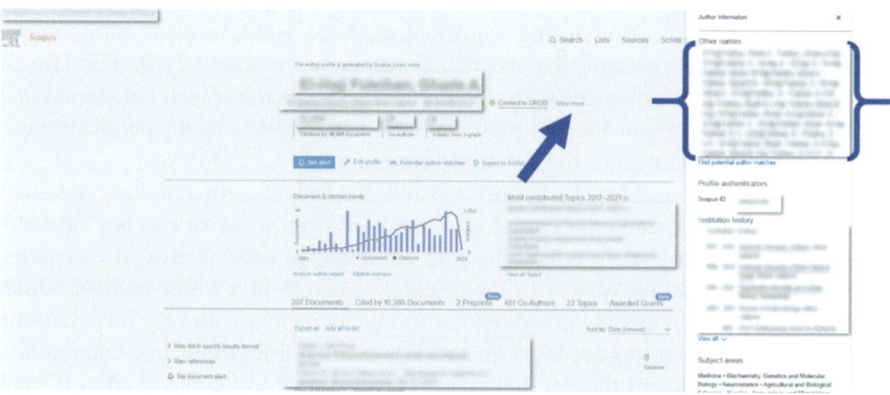

Fig. 5.8 Profile showing variations of names for the same researcher in her unique Scopus profile

Fig. 5.9 Scopus Author ID assigned under "Other IDs" in Scopus

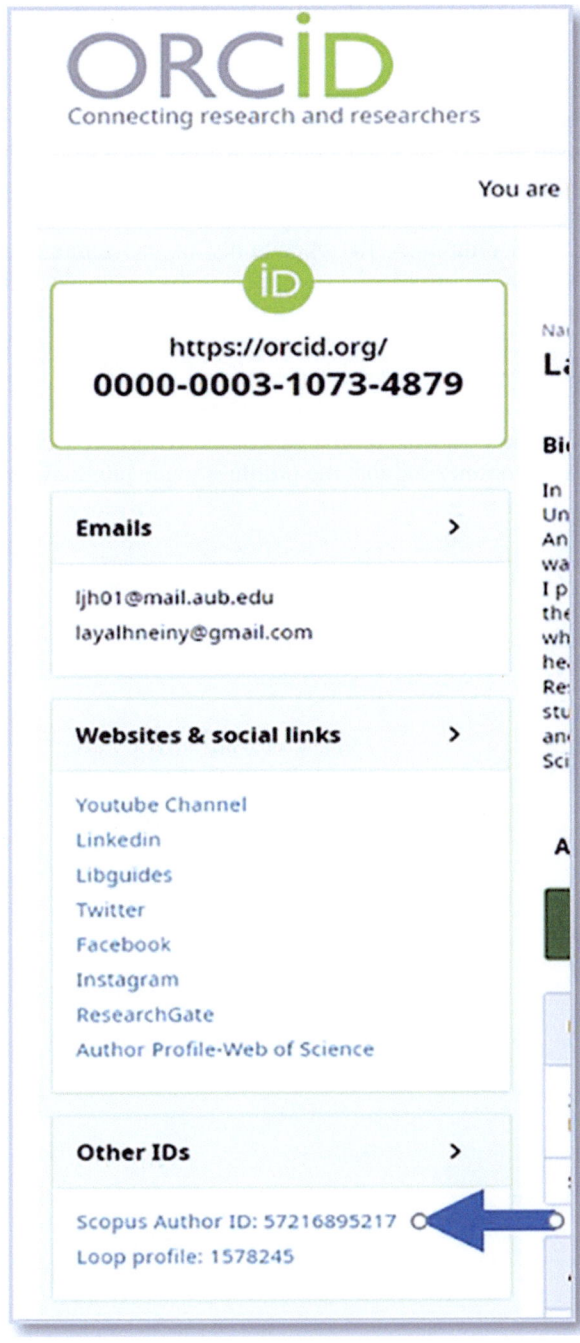

Web of Science: ResearcherID

Similar to Scopus Author ID, a unique identifier is provided by Clarivate via WoS citation analysis tool, ResearcherID. The "Researcher Profile" which displays the automatically assigned identifier ResearcherID, enables researchers to manage their list of publications, cited counts, citation percentile, co-authors, position as authors, and their h-index (see Fig. 5.10).

WoS eliminates the uncertainty of the author variant name-utilization issue. "Researcher profiles" can be associated with an ORCID profile, removing any ambiguity of the researcher's identity.

By clicking next to the ResearcherID number on "Share this profile" is a clear and easy way to help researchers market their profile by copying the URL provided and pasting it into the desired CV, blog, or website.

Privacy settings for the ResearcherID profile (see Fig. 5.11) are user controlled. It is recommended that the profile is made public for more visibility.

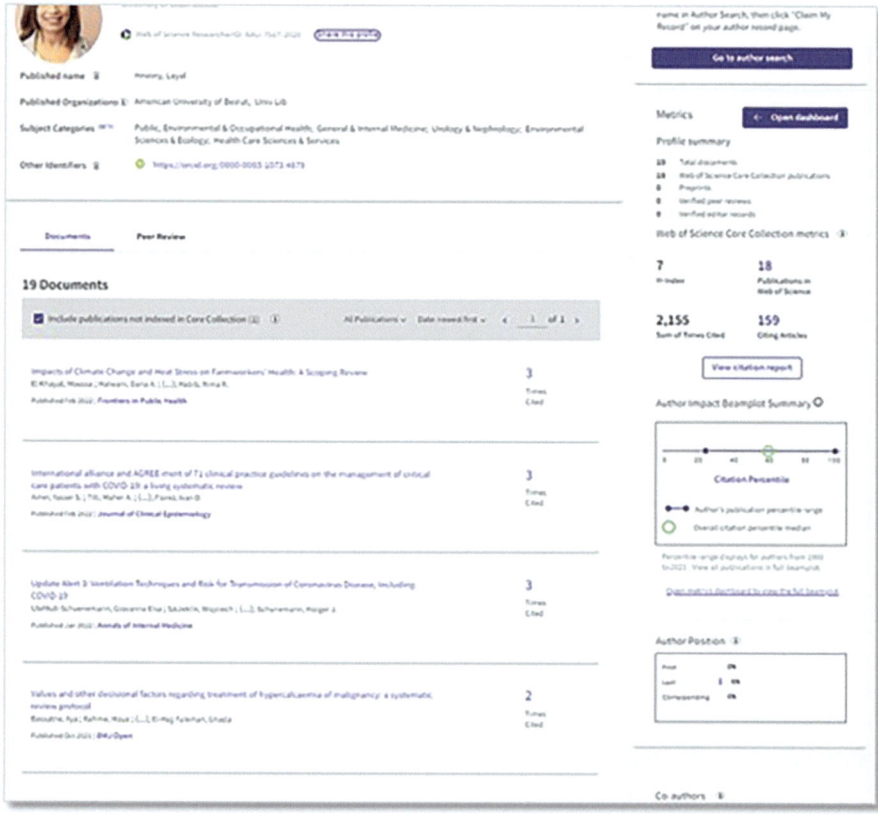

Fig. 5.10 The "Researcher Profile" features

5 Tools for Managing Your Digital Research Identity

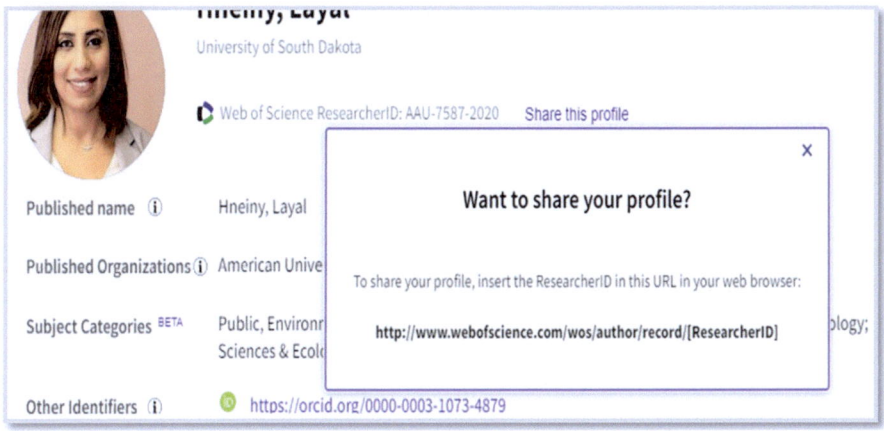

Fig. 5.11 In Researcher Profile: Where to find: WoS-ResearchID, sharing profile, published names, and the researcher's compliant ORCID profile

Google Scholar Profile

It is strongly suggested for researchers to establish a Google Scholar (GS) Profiles. First, it provides a simple way for the researcher to showcase their academic publications. Since the privacy settings are regulated by the user, making the profile public makes the it more visible. A second reason is that it provides the researcher with the ability to track who has cited their work. Thirdly, GS computes several citation metrics such as the citation count, h-index, and i-index and displays them on the GS profile (see Fig. 5.12).

While the formal h-index describes a researcher's publications over their entire career, it can also be described for a discrete period [15]. The h-index might differ among Scopus, WoS, and GS for the same researcher. It is usually higher in GS than in Scopus or WoS. A bibliometric analysis study done over a small selection of researcher working at a large public university revealed a high degree of similarity between both sources of citation information [16]. Yet, GS profile introduces another indicator, the i-10 index. This measurement can help scholars gauge their productivity. The i-10 index is described as the number of publications of an author with at least ten citations allowing scholars to distinguish their articles out of their publications that have received at least ten citations [17].

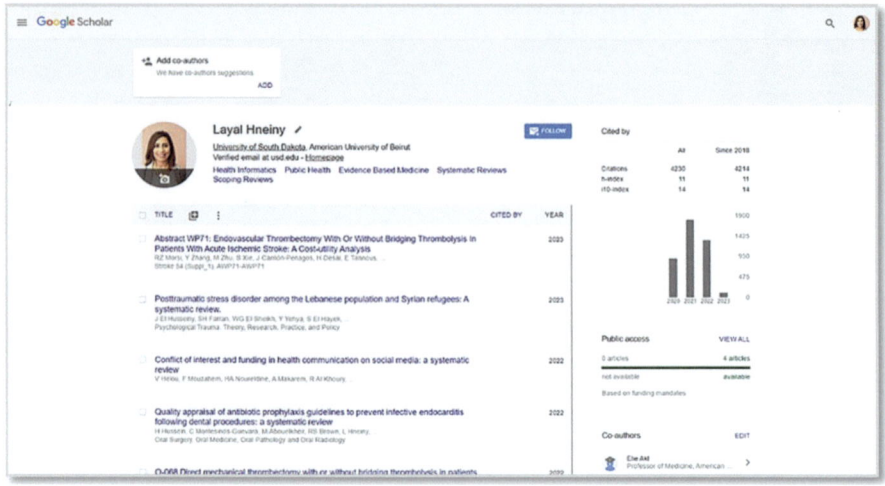

Fig. 5.12 A glimpse of Google Scholar Profile

ResearchGate: Between Traditional Metrics and Altmetrics

Along with traditional citation statistics, there are additional measurements calculated for the researcher drawn from other media platforms such as Twitter or X and Wikipedia (see Fig. 5.13).

5 Tools for Managing Your Digital Research Identity

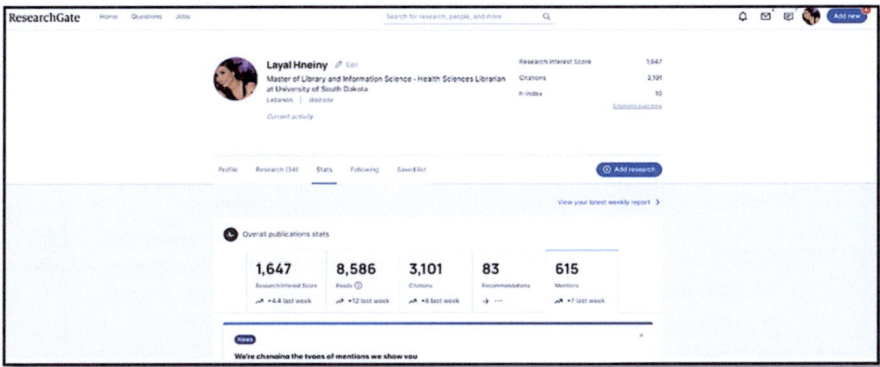

Fig. 5.13 In Researcher Profile: Where to find: Twitter. *This information is not always freely available to the public.*

Altmetrics Tools

News and information spreads quickly on social media. Altmetrics (https://www.altmetric.com) complements bibliometric studies by enabling a wider understanding of the real impact caused by scientific literature [18, 19]. Altmetics are powerful indicators that reveal what online communities are saying about your research in real time. News spreads worldwide within few seconds, so the moment the researcher's work is published Altmetrics can reveal how people are engaging in discussion about your work. Alternative metrics can assess the impact of the research by using a distinctive visualization tool that helps display a snapshot of a publication's online reach or influence by the "Altmetrics Badge."

The Altmetric Attention Score is highlighted indicating the impact of a research publication based on social media usage. The score represents a weighted count that takes into consideration the scanned [20] online sources including Twitter, blogs, news outlets, policy documents, Wikipedia, patents, and more to uncover the impact of the research.

Altmetrics is a powerful digital indicator that not only retrieves the "who" and "where" (which platform) but also the "what" is being said about the research (see Fig. 5.14). This creates a comprehensive instant feedback on the influence of research, which reflects the measure of societal impact. Altmetrics is a supplement to the traditional metrics, such as the h-index, that are tracked by waiting for citations from other's work.

To showcase the Altmetric Badge, scholars can click on the "Embed badge" button on the top right of the detailed Altmetric page and copy the html provided. A link can then be pasted to each of the publications in the author's CV, blog, or website.

Showcasing the Altmetric badge on your CV, blog, or website is a great way to manage your scholarly reputation. It can track the engagement of your published work, identifying the most operative outreach channel(s), identify collaborators and provide stakeholders with research outcomes that are grant funded.

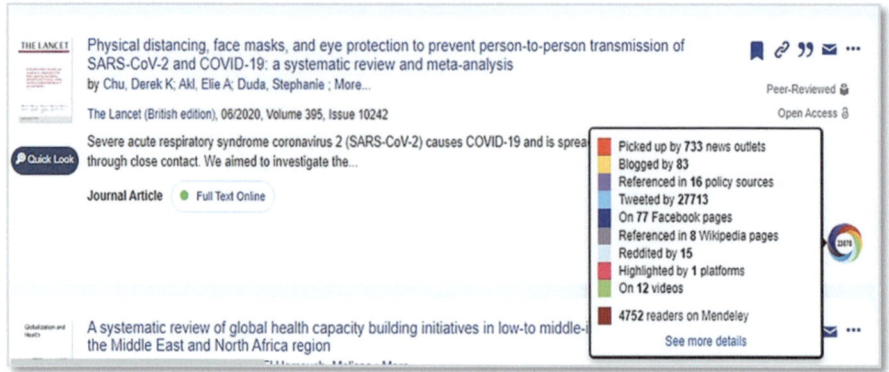

Fig. 5.14 How Altmetrics shows in Proquest Serials Solutions

Conclusion

It is crucial that researchers do not remain complacent, or these bibliometrics tools will not be able to provide information in which they were designed. This chapter discussed these tools in hopes to better manage a researcher's identity by providing clear access to digital profiles. These digital profiles can be used to promote a scholars work and make it accessible by acting as an outlet to researchers to promote the work [21]. It is beneficial for researchers to engage in social media networks that facilitate new means to manage their digital identity and disseminate their work.

References

1. Mauch JT, Azoury SC, Onyekaba G, Drolet BC, Janis JE, Fischer JP. Plastic surgery program leadership perspectives on doximity residency navigator rankings: do we need a better guide for prospective applicants? J Surg Educ. 2022;79:1076–81.
2. Walsh MN. Social media and cardiology. J Am Coll Cardiol. 2018;71:1044–7.
3. Lappalainen Y, Narayanan N. Harvesting publication data to the institutional repository from Scopus, Web of Science, Dimensions and Unpaywall using a custom R Script. J Acad Librariansh. 2023;49:102653. https://doi.org/10.1016/j.acalib.2022.102653.
4. ORCID and loop: a new researcher profile system integration. 2015. https://info.orcid.org/orcid-and-loop-a-new-researcher-profile-system-integration/. Accessed 14 Dec 2022.
5. Iqbal M, Ahmad M. Ranking and visualization of experts for communication using LinkedIn. In: Kohei A, Rahul B, Supriya K, editors. Advances in intelligent systems and computing, Future technologies conference (FTC). Cham: Springer; 2018. p. 1–12.
6. Kapoor N, Blumenthal DM, Smith SE, Ip IK, Khorasani R. Gender differences in academic rank of radiologists in US medical schools. Radiology. 2017;283:140–7. https://doi.org/10.1148/radiol.2016160950.
7. The professional medical network for physicians. 2023. https://www.doximity.com/about/company. Accessed 2 Dec 2023.

8. Sarli C. Establishing your author profile - tools for authors. 2023. https://beckerguides.wustl.edu/authors/authorname. Accessed 15 Jan 2023.
9. Meade PJ, Amin SJ, Stamm MA, Mulcahey MK. Doximity orthopaedic surgery program rankings are associated with academic productivity. JBJS Open Access. 2023;68:e22.00081. https://doi.org/10.2106/JBJS.OA.22.00081.
10. Leung SJ, Chiang BJ, Roseman JT, Klausner A. The utility of social media on urology residency doximity rankings. Cureus. 2022;14:e29666. https://doi.org/10.7759/cureus.29666.
11. Lee J, Oh S, Dong H, Wang F, Burnett G. Motivations for self-archiving on an academic social networking site: a study on researchgate. JASIST. 2019;70:563–74. https://doi.org/10.1002/asi.24138.
12. Liu XZ, Fang H. Which academic papers do researchers tend to feature on ResearchGate? Inform Res. 2018;23:25.
13. Quaia E, Vernuccio F. The H index myth: a form of fanaticism or a simple misconception? MDPI. 2022;8:1241–3. https://doi.org/10.3390/tomography8030102.
14. Shah FA, Jawaid SA. The h-index: an indicator of research and publication output. Pak J Med Sci. 2023;39(2):315–6. https://doi.org/10.12669/pjms.39.2.7398.
15. Shiah E, Heiman AJ, Ricci JA. Evaluation of the i10-index in plastic surgery research and its correlation with altmetric attention scores and traditional author bibliometrics: an evaluation of a single journal. Indian J Plast Surg. 2023;56(1):68–73. https://doi.org/10.1055/s-0043-1760827.
16. Dunaway D. Bibliometrics for faculty evaluation: a statistical comparison of h-indexes generated using Google Scholar and Web of Science data. Codex. 2019;5:18–29.
17. Aithal P. Comparative study of various research indices used to measure quality of research publications. IJAASR. 2017;2:81–9. https://doi.org/10.5281/zenodo.569763.
18. Gontijo MCA, de Araujo RF. Academic impact and on-line attention of papers on artificial intelligence in health field: bibliometric and altmetric analysis. Encontros Bibli-Revista Eletronica De Biblioteconomia E Ciencia Da Informacao. 2021;26:1–21. https://doi.org/10.5007/1518-2924.2021.e76249.
19. Powell A, Bevan V, Brown C, Lewis WG. Altmetric versus bibliometric perspective regarding publication impact and force. World J Surg. 2018;42:2745–56. https://doi.org/10.1007/s00268-018-4579-9.
20. Altmetric: about our data. https://www.altmetric.com/about-our-data/the-donut-and-score/.2023. Accessed 4 Oct 2022.
21. Iglesias-Garcia M, Gonzalez-Diaz C, Codina L. A study of student and university teaching staff presence on ResearchGate and Academia.edu in Spain. In: Freire FC, Araujo XR, VAM F, Garcia XL, editors. Media and metamedia management, Advances in intelligent systems and computing. Cham: Springer; 2017. p. 509–15.

Chapter 6
Author Metrics

Kyle James Downey

Introduction

Managing a research identity in the era of digitization allows for the opportunity of researchers to increase their visibility and research impact throughout the world. In this scholarly ecosystem, the use of systematic measures like bibliometrics has allowed for the quantification of researcher productivity to be broadcasted to a wider academic community. These metrics or indices allow for the evaluation of the impact of research that has been conducted and published by an individual author which can lead to further advances in their relative field of research.

Publication metrics such as the journal impact factor are being used to make important decisions with regards to the process of hiring, promotions, tenure, and research funding. Author metrics, such as the h-index, are also being used to make these critical and career defining decisions. These quantitative ways of measuring publication and citation counts can inform others about research productivity, collaboration, and the impact of individual authors, teams, and universities. Although bibliometric indicators like the h-index are the most widely used, they certainly have their shortcomings and limitations. Used as a complement alongside the more traditional qualitative evaluation approach such as peer review, will give authors a more well-rounded understanding of their academic publication impact [1].

In this chapter we will be discussing the use of author and alternative metrics. Author metrics are being used widely throughout academia to evaluate an author's research impact and output. There are several different methods of measuring and evaluating one's impact and no one specific indicator will provide the full picture. Understanding how these metrics work, or how they are meant to work, will give

K. J. Downey (✉)
Nursing & Health Sciences Librarian, Seton Hall University, Nutley, NJ, USA
e-mail: kyle.downey@shu.edu

© The Author(s), under exclusive license to Springer Nature Switzerland AG 2023
M. R. Dreker, K. J. Downey (eds.), *Building Your Academic Research Digital Identity*, https://doi.org/10.1007/978-3-031-50317-7_6

researchers the tools to create and forge new opportunities in their field including additional grant funding as well as new hiring and promotion initiatives.

The indices discussed in this chapter will include the h-index, g-index, e-index, I-10 index, and the Author Impact Factor (AIF). The purpose of this chapter is to inform researchers about author metrics so that they can become aware of the evaluative techniques being applied to their scientific output as well as improve their scientific impact. This chapter will not be able to inform researchers on all the metrics that are available as there are several dozen that are being used. This chapter will not go into the mathematical interpretation and computation detail of each index as that is beyond the scope and message of this book. While this chapter gives researchers a glimpse into what these metrics are and how they are used, we must understand that no single metric or parameter defines someone's scientific and publishing excellence. There are limitations and shortcomings to these metrics that will be discussed.

This chapter will also discuss the use of alternative metrics, or altmetrics. While author metrics are being used as the traditional method of measuring academic success, altmetrics are allowing authors to move beyond the traditional printed journal page to measure their impact. We will discuss what they are and how they complement traditional academic measures.

Author Metrics

The traditional way of evaluating one's quality and impact of research is through the publication list of a scholar. As competition for funding only increases, quantifying the research output of academics is becoming more important in determining one's publishing impact [2]. Knowing the scientific impact of a scholar is even becoming necessary as institutions will look for these metrics during times of hiring a new faculty member, the promotion of employees and the application of research grants.

To measure the publishing impact of a scholar, numerous citation metrics have been proposed to the academic community. Working alongside the continuation of the qualitative peer review process of evaluation, these metrics can provide valuable information for reporting the impact of publication output.

The quantification of research productivity by indices like the h-index and others will be used increasingly as a benchmark for performance of a researcher [3]. Therefore, as a researcher, it will be beneficial to understand what these indices' purposes are, how they differ from one another in their scoring and their limitations. As we continue to use bibliometrics like the h-index to systematically measure research output, we also must remember that no metric will give us a complete reflection of one's publication productivity.

The H-Index

The h-index is the most widely known, discussed, and used index for measuring academic author productivity. It is the most sophisticated and intricate measure among the various other author metrics since it accounts for both the quality and the quantity of a researcher's publications. The concept was introduced by Jorge Hirsch in 2005 as a way to conduct a "simple and useful way to characterize the scientific output of a researcher" [1], by quantifying the cumulative impact of an author's scientific publication [4].

Mathematically the index can simply be broken down as the largest number of h papers with at least h number of citations. A simple example of this would be if a researcher has an h-index score of 25, that means he or she has published at least 25 articles which have been cited at least 25 times each. The h-index according to Hirsch gives us "an estimate of the importance, significance, and broad impact of a scientist's cumulative research contributions" [5]. While Hirsch's research on the h-index was concentrated on physicists, he reasoned that the h-index would be useful for other scientific disciplines as well.

The h-index was a breakthrough in the scientific community because of the way it accesses and evaluates scientific research output in such a simplistic way. It received a positive acceptance in the scientific community because it provided a solution of combining the number of published papers and the number of citations in a noncomplex fashion [6]. This combination of simultaneously measuring both the productivity and the impact of an author by including the quality and quantity of one's publishing activity is why it has been popular amongst the field of several bibliometric indexes.

Using the H-Index

As an author your h-index score is used as a metric of your scientific output by considering the maximum number of papers which also have at least the same number of citations. If you have an h-index score of 10, that means that you have at least 10 published articles that have each been cited at least 10 times [3, 6].

The h-index does not use complicated mathematical operations of data, such as multiplying or dividing publications and citations, to create an index score. Rather, the h-index score is obtained as a result of a process [7]. Hirsch considered papers with at least h citations as the most impactful publications in one's career [2].

The h-index provides us with an alternative to counting the total number of citations, as well as an alternative to counting the number of highly cited publications of a particular author [8]. Because of this, many authors agree that the h-index is insensitive to both highly cited publications but also lowly cited and uncited publications too.

Limitations of the H-Index

In the world of bibliometrics, the h-index is considered a "classical bibliometric indicator" [9] or even a "mainstream bibliometric indicator" [10]. It continues to be widely used by researchers as the main way to score their scientific output. The h-index, however, has been routinely criticized since its initial publication back in 2005. There has been continued academic debate along with several publications on using alternative impact metrics to fairly assess a scholars publication output, regardless of the field they are in or other limiting factors.

Calculations for the h-index are insensitive based on a number of factors which include: incomparability between disciplines, article types, highly cited items, total citations, self-citations, number of co-authors, research funding, and countries. It is difficult to compare researchers with different career spans because it is a simple function of productivity and impact, therefore authors with longer careers will have higher scores. Meanwhile authors with a shorter career span begin their careers with less publications and citations and therefore will have a lower score. Younger researchers may also have to contend with heavier workloads, such as teaching responsibilities, that may interfere or hinder their ability to publish. Essentially, authors with a longer career and more publications will always have a higher h-index score.

Authors with a lesser number of publications and citations may also be tempted to inflate their scores with irrelevant self-citations. Self-citing one's work could lead to the possibility of increasing one's h-index score annually by 1 [4]. Lastly, the h-index score does not consider or provide different values based on author contributions, therefore a researcher does not have to be a solo author in order to increase their h-index score.

Since its introduction, the h-index has been the most widely accepted author metric score in the scientific community. It was developed as an alternative to the journal impact factor as an attempt to measure both the scientific productivity and the scientific impact of a researcher. It has helped successful researchers obtain grants, employment, and world recognition within their fields of work.

It is important to emphasize that the h-index score isn't and shouldn't be the only metric used to measure your research impact [8]. It is essential to understand that research impact and productivity is more complex than what a single number can provide. It is, therefore, desirable and also practical to use multiple bibliometric indicators in order to establish your research impact. Discussed below are some additional author metrics that are widely used in academia to measure author impact.

Additional Author Metrics

g-Index

The g-index was introduced in 2006 by Leo Egghe for measuring and comparing the output of scientific researchers. It was proposed as an improvement of the h-index as its purpose is to give more weight to highly cited papers [11]. It is calculated based on the distribution of citations received by a researcher's publications, such that:

> [Given a set of articles] ranked in decreasing order of the number of citations that they received, the g-index is the (unique) largest number such that the top g articles received (together) at least g2 citations [12].

It was proposed by Egghe as the answer to an h-index limitation: once an article belongs to the H top class, it is no longer important whether that article is continually cited or not. The g-index modifies the h-index by dealing with the high performance of the top articles and counting their number of citations regardless if the article is already at the top class [13]. Essentially, the g-index gives more weight to highly cited papers, whereas the h-index is insensitive to it.

A g-index of 10 means that a researcher has published at least 10 articles that combined have received at least 100 citations. This means that if a researcher has published 10 articles, 5 of which received no citations while the other five having 55, 20, 15, 7, 3 citations would have a g-index of 10, regardless of if 5 of their papers haven't been cited.

The g-index may be more acceptable for researchers who are less likely to obtain high values of the h-index because the weighing of citations received by the documents is considered in the g-index calculation and the g-index for a given researchers not limited by the total number of publications [14].

However, just like the h-index, there are limitations to the g-index. The existence of different types of documents with different impacts; the problems with self-citations, and the inability to compare researchers from different fields of science and academia remain as limitations [15].

e-Index

The e-index was proposed by Chun-Ting Zhang to help distinguish researchers who have excessive total citations, with a focus in favor of highly cited researchers [16]. The overall aim of the metric is to differentiate between scientists with similar h-indices but have different citation patterns [17]. The e-index also helps calculate the ignored excess citations that a researcher may be receiving over the h-index. Using the e-index in conjunction with the h-index allows researchers to get a more accurate and fair comparison of their academic output with researchers with a similar h-index score [13]. However, like the h-index, the e-index alone is not the preferred tool to use for researchers with few publications, citations, or is new to their field [18].

i10-Index

The i10-index is a scholarly metric that measures the number of publications with 10 or more citations. The index was founded in 2011 by Google as a way to help measure the productivity of a scholar. In order for an author to have their scholarly research included in the i10-index, the author must first create a public Google Scholar profile. After creating a Google Scholar profile, a researcher will then add their publications to their account to establish an i10 score [19].

To calculate an i10 score, an author must have a minimum of 10 citations per publication. Fr example, if an author has 10 published papers, but only 7 of which have 10 or more citations, then their i10 score would be a 7. Of course, there are limitations to using the i10-index as a measure of one's productivity. One limitation is that it is only calculated and found within Google Scholar. Another limitation is that the i10-index may not be an appropriate distinguishing factor for scholars with high citation counts [20]. Despite those minor limitations, the i10-index is one of the easiest author metrics to understand and calculate.

Author Impact Factor (AIF)

The AIF was introduced in 2014 as an extension of the Impact Factor (IF) for publications, but with a focus on authors. The AIF is calculated similarly to the IF, however, instead of focusing on where papers are published, the AIF considers the publications of an author by monitoring the evolution of their performance and scholarly output. It is calculated by the number of citations to an author's articles, which are published in a certain year, divided by the number of the evaluated author's articles in the previous 5-year period [4].

The AIF, unlike other indexes, is considered dynamic, in that it follows the evolution of the impact of a scholar. This allows the index to identify when a scholar is either in a rising or declining phase of their career. It also incentivizes authors to do high quality research by averaging a number of citations received by all papers published by an author in a given time window. Their AIF score will be high if those papers are well cited, however low-quality work will keep their score down [21].

The AIF calculation is similar to that of the IF, so it can easily be implemented in most bibliographic databases for assessment. It follows the evolution of a researcher's career, which might be decisive for organizations during the hiring process. And unlike the h-index, the AIF considers the quality of a paper rather than just how many or where a paper is published.

Measuring Tools for Authors and Collaborators

Bibliographic databases, often referred to in this context as profiling platforms, allow for researchers and authors to add their publication and citation content to increase their visibility of their research output and impact. These profile platforms have become increasingly important for scholars because not only does it allow them to display their academic and research accomplishments, but it also allows them to collaborate with fellow researchers on additional research, as well as compete for grant funding and promotional opportunities [4].

Widely accepted as the most comprehensive data source for publication metadata and citation metrics are profiling platforms Scopus (Elseview) and Web of Science (WoS) (Clarivate). Scopus and WoS have been used extensively to evaluate research productivity across different academic disciplines for well over two decades. These profiling platforms provide authors with their estimated h-index score along with other author and journal publication metrics. Along with Google Scholar, these profiling platforms are important for scholars to demonstrate their academic impact to a wider audience (see Chap. 5).

Web of Science

Web of Science (WoS) is a multidisciplinary database that can be used to gather and organize author information for the purpose of evaluating one's author impact. Scholars can use WoS to perform a basic analysis of their research outputs and to find metrics such as their h-index, overall citations, and publications. They can also export lists of their publications and citations. Like all databases, WoS does not include all articles published, but its selection of journals are highly respected and useful for citation analysis.

The WoS Citation Reports provides statistical information about an author's publishing output and the citations the author's work has received. It can be used to discern patterns, find an h-index, and get a complete picture of the publishing and citation history of an individual author. Researchers can also use the Analyze Results feature in WoS to identify citation metrics and trends relating to authors, publications, institutions, and collaborations.

WoS has number of bibliographic tools that allow researchers to create citation reports in order to create a breakdown of times cited by year, h-index score, average citation per year, and the sum of non-self-citations for the author. A major limitation to WoS is that this is not a free product. One must purchase a license or work for an institution that has the subscribed package.

Scopus

Scopus is bibliographic citation database containing peer-reviewed journals, scientific literature, books, and conference proceedings. Scopus is owned by the publisher Elsevier and is available online with a subscription (since 2004). Researchers can conduct searches for authors in Scopus by using an author's Open Researcher and Contributor ID (ORCID) or an author's last name, initials or first name, and their affiliation [22]. Author metrics are automatically generated, and a Scopus ID is created when the author gets at least one citation indexed within Scopus. Once indexed, an author has the ability to track and analyze their citation data including their h-index score [23].

The Scopus Author Profile allows the database to group and track publications by a specific author, attempting to group publications under the correct profile. Scopus allows authors to update and correct their profile, which is especially important if multiple authors have the same name. Authors have the ability to update their entries of their publications, track new citations of their work, review research metrics based on their publication record and link their profile to their ORCID record (see Fig. 6.1).

There are of course limitations to using Scopus as the only way to track author citation records. Scopus has a limited timeline of content, going back to only 1996 for many of its records. This may misrepresent author profiles who have a longer established academic career with highly cited works. There are also technical errors that occasionally occur within Scopus due to the automatic processing of the data. This may lead to more than one identifier being used for the same author [23]. Despite these flaws, Scopus is an excellent tool that can help track your publication impact in a clean and efficient manner. An author may have to regularly monitor

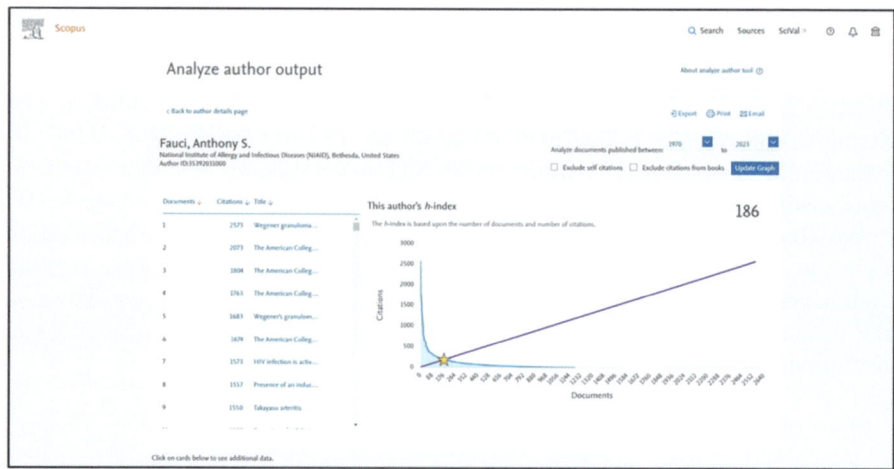

Fig. 6.1 Scopus Author output example using Dr. Fauci's profile

their profile so that everything has been captured sufficiently, but establishing a Scopus profile is a great way to track an author's citations.

Google Scholar Citations

Google Scholar is a free and easily accessible platform that contains many publications beyond journal articles, such as books, reports, patents, presentations, posters, and other materials [24]. In 2011, Google launched Google Scholar Citations; a free platform for global citation tracking which functions as a free alternative to WoS and Scopus. An author can create a free profile on Google Scholar which will allow them to add their affiliation(s), research interests, publication list, and citations. With a Google Scholar profile established, an author can track who is citing their publications as well as the ability to track their citation metrics using popular indices such as the h-index and the i10-index (see Fig. 6.2).

Establishing a profile in Google Scholar Citations can benefit researchers who are in early in their career. Unlike Scopus or WoS, Google Scholar benefits the younger, less established scholar, especially one that is in the Social Sciences or the Humanities because Google Scholar is indexing more journals and more publication types than other databases. The service indexes across a wide range of sources from academic disciplines including academic publishers, professional societies, online repositories, universities, and other academic websites.

There are limitations to using Google Scholar Citations. As Google crawls the web creating citation connections, sometimes it may create duplicate records for the same publication. The lack of filtering out poor quality work, self-citation boosting, and the indexing of predatory sources are also some of the main limitations for Google Scholar [25].

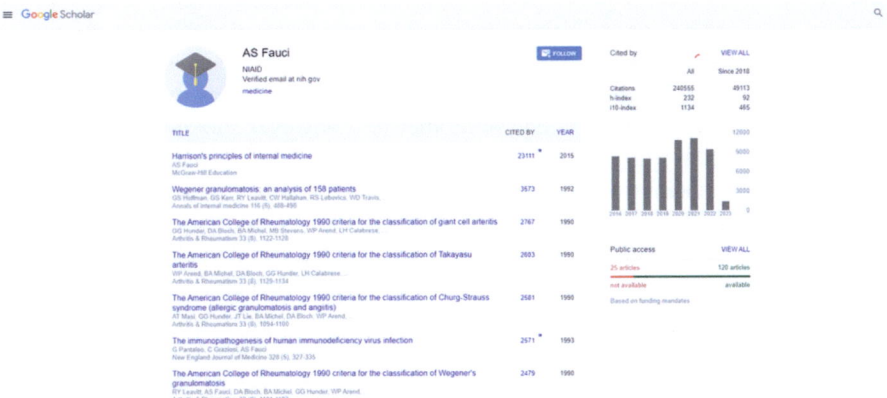

Fig. 6.2 Google Scholar Profile

With those limitations in mind, Google Scholar Citations is still an effective platform that allows authors to track their citations of their own publications over time. Using citation metrics and easy-to-read graphs, authors, especially one's early in their career, will be able to build their own profile to track their citations and follow research themes for further collaboration. It is a free tool, unlike WoS and Scopus, and its coverage extends into the Social Sciences and Humanities disciplines.

Summary of Traditional Author Metrics

Author-level metrics, and the profiling platforms that store and display that information, serve as a benchmark for scholarly productivity within academia. Research in academia will only continue to get more competitive as scholars contend for research funding as well as promotions and raises. That is why it is important for authors to establish themselves on author profile platforms and understand the use of author metrics to develop their discoverability and impact [3].

It is important to also understand that while author-level indices can provide compelling narratives of academic impact, no single metric is sufficient or comprehensive enough to accurately reflect the scope of scholarly activities (see Table 6.1). While these metrics help encourage healthy and constructive competition amongst scholars, we must also remember that measuring and evaluating one's research productivity is a complex procedure that no one single metric can portray [26]. The approach to measure one's author-level output based on one score should not be practiced [27] as it does provide the full story or efforts of an author's impact or influence.

Alternative Metrics

Author-level metrics such as the h-index and i10-index have been seen as the standard method of quantifying scholarly impact that an author has made within their academic community. Traditional bibliometrics, however, do not represent the impact authors may have beyond the sphere of academia. It does not take into account the role social media and other media platforms have done to disseminate knowledge [28]. In recent years, alternative metrics or altmetrics, have become another option for assessing scholarly impact through a societal lens. In this section we will briefly talk about what defines altmetrics and its benefits and disadvantages of its scholarly research impact.

Altmetrics are defined as web-based metrics with an emphasis on social media outlets as a source of data [29]. They are relatively new, despite growing in popularity, so it shouldn't be a surprise if most authors are unfamiliar with it. With the way social media is used today, altmetrics can help us to understand how an article

Table 6.1 Strengths and limitations of author-level metrics

Metrics	Strengths	Limitations
h-index	Easy to calculate, provides a single number which is easy to understand, reflects productivity, and is useful for comparing highly productive researchers	Favors researchers with longer careers, varies across different disciplines due to different citation practices, can be manipulated by self-citations, does not differentiate between the contribution of co-authors
g-index	Easy to calculate, gives more weight to highly cited items, allows the comparison of authors in different disciplines, tracks author's impact over time	Does not consider quality of individual publications, but rather accounts for all publications being of high quality, can be manipulated by self-citations, dependent on the average number of citations for all published papers
e-index	Easy to calculate, emphases on highly cited publications; helps distinguish highly productive authors with identical h-index scores but differing total citation counts, measures long-term impact	Biased towards senior researchers with multiple publications and citation counts, discipline-specific, manipulation by citations and citation stacking, ignores co-authorship
l10-index	Easy to calculate, not influenced by only highly cited publications, calculated through Google Scholar which makes the data publicly available	May still not capture the full range of a researcher's citation impact, subject to self-citation, lack of quality control
Author Impact Factor	Focus on citation activity in 5-year increments, captures trends and variations of the impact of the scientific output of researchers in time	Capturing citation activity in smaller increments may not demonstrate the impact of authors in slowly developing disciplines

performs on the web outside of the traditional citation counts. Altmetrics covers other impact factors of an article including how many times an article has been viewed, how many full-text downloads, social media likes, and mentioning's on blogs or the news [30]. Additionally, altmetrics involves how many times an article has been added to a citation management software system such as Mendeley or Zotero.

One goal of altmetrics is to provide a comprehensive and timely view of the impact of research. Traditionally, it takes years for citation counts to build up, which can be a major disservice to younger, less established authors. Altmetrics not only demonstrates the impact of research in a timelier manner, but it is also useful for assessing the impact of newer forms of research output such as datasets, software, and preprints. These kinds of research outputs are not found in peer-reviewed journals.

Data aggregators such as Altmetric.com and PlumX Altmetrics Dashboard (Plum Analytics), offer several tools and services that provide altmetric data [31]. PlumX is a research metrics and analysis platform that measures the impact of research output across several different channels. PlumX uses a variety of traditional citation-based metrics, as well alternative metrics, to evaluate the impact of a research from research articles, conference proceedings and book chapters.

Altmetric.com was founded in 2011 in London, UK. It is a web-based platform that provides alternative metrics for measuring the impact of scholarly publications through the tracking of online engagement and interaction, that goes beyond what traditional citation-based metrics can represent. Sources such as social media, policy documents, mainstream media and online reference managers are collected by Altmetric to develop newer versions of impact metrics.

Users may see Altmetric widgets embedded within databases, e-journal platforms, and even institutional repositories. The widget, also known as a donut badge, allows users to visit the details of the research output through a variety of different colors that represent a different source of attention. This includes sources from the news, blogs, Twitter (X), Facebook, LinkedIn, Reddit, YouTube, and Wikipedia. The colors are affected and will change depending on what sources the research output receives attention from. This means that if a donut badge is predominately red, then the research output has received a lot of media attention [32]. Ultimately the widget is a useful tool for researchers, publishers, and institutions for tracking online conversations regarding their research impact [33].

PlumX gathers research metrics into five separate categories which include Citations, Usage, Captures, Mentions, and Social Media [34]. The aggregation of this data from those categories provides a comprehensive view of the impact of research output that traditional citation-based metrics cannot capture. Academic institutions, research organizations, and individual researchers can use PlumX to help track and evaluate the impact of their research, identify gaps in knowledge, establish collaborations, and benchmark their performance against similar researchers in their field.

There are of course limitations to altmetrics, as they are vulnerable to manipulation and their lasting impact hasn't been fully studied. Altmetric data is collected via web-based media platforms and because of this it can be subjected to gaming and artificial bias [35]. Individuals may use these limitations to influence the number of times their research content is being accessed and used.

There is also a stronger emphasis in the academic disciplines of science and medicine which makes interdisciplinary comparisons of altmetric data limited. Ultimately, more research still needs to be conducted to understand the true impact of altmetrics, especially with regards to its use for faculty tenure, promotions, grant applications and overall scholarly research impact.

Altmetrics measures the attention and impact of scholarly work by analyzing the number of times it has been viewed, downloaded, social media mentions, likes, bookmarks and in addition to online citation reference managers. The goal is to provide a more comprehensive and timely view of the impact of research that reaches beyond the traditional citation count. While bringing new insight into the impact of scholarly work, limitations exist including biases, manipulation, limited coverage, inconsistent data, and lack of context [35]. Altmetrics should be used in conjunction, rather than replace traditional metrics, to provide a more comprehensive and well-rounded understanding of the impact of scholarly work.

Conclusion

In academia, the use of scholarly metrics, specifically author metrics, has become the standard of practice for measuring one's research impact. Indices such as the h-index are still being actively used while other indices are being developed to measure different forms of impact. Though these indices are very helpful to academics and researchers who are seeking tenure, promotion, or funding, it must be understood that no metric number gives the full picture of one's knowledge, research, or expertise. Many disciplines outside of the sciences and health sciences may not benefit from a h-index or similar metric score.

Altmetrics takes a different approach to measuring one's research output. By incorporating non-traditional sources like social media, the news, blog posts and citation management data, altmetrics can demonstrate how one's research and expertise is being disseminated and used outside of the traditional journal citation count. This can widely benefit both the researcher as well as the institution they work for by circulating their research to a broader audience without the barriers of paywalls or journal subscriptions.

If you are either new to the field of research, or you have several publications under your belt, it is strongly recommended that you take some time to learn about these indices. If you work for an academic institution, see whether they have Scopus or WoS so that you can keep track of your scholarly metrics. Work alongside a librarian or another colleague to make sure your information is up to date and accurate. If you don't belong to an academic institution, you can still use Google Scholar to keep track of your work as well. There may be limitations of relying on just author metrics to measure one's research impact, but currently, aside from altmetrics, it is the only way to measure impact formally.

References

1. Maggio LA, Jeffrey A, Haustein S, Samuel A. Becoming metrics literate: an analysis of brief videos that teach about the h-index. PLoS One. 2022;17(5):1–16.
2. Bornmann L, Marx W. The h-index as a research performance indicator. Eur Sci Ed. 2011;37(3):77–80.
3. Carpenter CR, Cone DC, Sarli CC. Using publication metrics to highlight academic productivity and research impact. Acad Emerg Med. 2014;21(10):1160–72.
4. Gasparyan AY, Yessirkepov M, Duisenova A, Trukhachev VI, Kostyukova EI, Kitas GD. Researcher and author impact metrics: variety, value, and context. J Korean Med Sci. 2018;33(18):e139.
5. Hirsch JE. An index to quantify an individual's scientific research output. Proc Natl Acad Sci U S A. 2005;102(46):16569–72.
6. Kaptay G. The k-index is introduced to replace the h-index to evaluate better the scientific excellence of individuals. Heliyon. 2020;6(7):e04415.
7. Egghe L, Rousseau R. The h-index formalism. Scientometrics. 2021;126(7):6137–45.

8. Waltman L, van Eck NJ. The inconsistency of the h-index. J Am Soc Inf Sci Technol. 2012;63(2):406–15.
9. Fraumann G, Mutz R. The h-index. In: Handbook bibliometrics. Berlin: Walter de Gruyter GmbH & Co KG; 2021. p. 169–201.
10. Costas R, Franssen T. Reflections around 'the cautionary use' of the h-index: response to Teixeira da Silva and Dobránszki. Scientometrics. 2018;115(2):1125–30.
11. Woeginger GJ. An axiomatic analysis of Egghe's g-index. J Informet. 2008;2(4):364–8.
12. Egghe L. Theory and practise of the g-index. Scientometrics. 2006;69(1):131–52.
13. Roldan-Valadez E, Salazar-Ruiz SY, Ibarra-Contreras R, Rios C. Current concepts on bibliometrics: a brief review about impact factor, Eigenfactor score, CiteScore, SCImago Journal Rank, Source-Normalised Impact per Paper, H-index, and alternative metrics. Ir J Med Sci. 2019;188(3):939–51.
14. Costas R, Bordons M. Is g-index better than h-index? An exploratory study at the individual level. Scientometrics. 2008;77(2):267–88.
15. Vinkler P. Eminence of scientists in the light of the h-index and other scientometric indicators. J Inf Sci. 2007;33(4):481–91.
16. Zhang CT. The e-index, complementing the h-index for excess citations. PLoS One. 2009;4(5):e5429.
17. Zhang CT. Relationship of the h-index, g-index, and e-index. J Am Soc Inf Sci Technol. 2010;61(3):625–8.
18. Dodson MV. Citation analysis: maintenance of h-index and use of e-index. Biochem Biophys Res Commun. 2009;387(4):625–6.
19. Dhamdhere SN. Cumulative citations index, h-index and i10-index (research metrics) of an educational institute: a case study. IJLIS. 2018;10(1):1–9.
20. Teixeira da Silva JA. The i100-index, i1000-index and i10,000-index: expansion and fortification of the Google Scholar h-index for finer-scale citation descriptions and researcher classification. Scientometrics. 2021;126(4):3667–72.
21. Pan RK, Fortunato S. Author impact factor: tracking the dynamics of individual scientific impact. Sci Rep. 2014;4(1):4880.
22. Stuart A, Faucette SP, Thomas WJ. Author impact metrics in communication sciences and disorder research. J Speech Lang Hear Res. 2017;60(9):2704.
23. Gasparyan AY, Nurmashev B, Yessirkepov M, Endovitskiy DA, Voronov AA, Kitas GD. Researcher and author profiles: opportunities, advantages, and limitations. J Korean Med Sci. 2017;32(11):1749–56.
24. About Google Scholar. https://scholar.google.com/intl/en/scholar/about.html.
25. Falagas ME, Pitsouni EI, Malietzis GA, Pappas G. Comparison of PubMed, Scopus, Web of Science, and Google Scholar: strengths and weaknesses. FASEB J. 2008;22(2):338–42.
26. Yelamanchi R, Agrawal H, Gupta N. Author level metrics and academic productivity. Int J Surg. 2021;90:105965.
27. Ali MJ. Forewarned is forearmed: the h-index as a scientometric. Semin Ophthalmol. 2021;36(1–2):1–1.
28. Bajwa SJS, Mehdiratta L. From traditional bibliometrics to altmetrics: socialising the research metrics. Indian J Anaesth. 2021;65(12):849–52.
29. Shema H, Bar-Ilan J, Thelwall M. Do blog citations correlate with a higher number of future citations? Research blogs as a potential source for alternative metrics. J Assoc Inf Sci Technol. 2014;65(5):1018–27.
30. Olff M. Are we happy with the impact factor? Eur J Psychotraumatol. 2014;5(1):26084.
31. Ortega JL. Altmetrics data providers: a meta-analysis review of the coverage of metrics and publication. Profesional de la información. 2020;29(1) https://doi.org/10.3145/epi.2020.ene.07.
32. The donut and Altmetric Attention Score. Altmetric. 2015. https://www.altmetric.com/about-our-data/the-donut-and-score/.

33. Finch T, O'Hanlon N, Dudley SP. Tweeting birds: online mentions predict future citations in ornithology. R Soc Open Sci. 2017;4(11):171371.
34. About PlumX metrics - plum analytics. https://plumanalytics.com/learn/about-metrics/.
35. Thelwall M. The pros and cons of the use of altmetrics in research assessment. Sch Assess Rep. 2020;2(1):2.

Chapter 7
Additional Measures to Establish Your Digital Identity

Plato Smith

Introduction

The National Science Foundation (NSF) will mandate to only use SciENcv for the biographical sketch in preparation of new proposals submitted or due on or after October 23, 2023 [1]. This makes it evident to adopt added measures to establish your academic digital identity. Added measures include the development of a personal website of your academic career online that is institution-independent and vendor-agnostic (external or independent platform) to enable sustainability over the life of your academic career.

Author profiles included as part of vendor products can be ephemeral limited to institution, product, or vendor. However, an independent personal website of your academic career, including conferences and research projects, developed, maintained, and sustained by you is far more maintainable than your institutional support. Research project websites supported by the institution, funder, or vendor are not guaranteed. You must support your website.

On February 14, 2023, a Research Governance Officer—Open Research from De Montfort University in Leicester, England started an interesting thread titled "How does your institution support websites beyond project life?" on the RESEARCH-DATAMAN@JISCMAIL.AC.UK listserv. The questions posted to the international data management listserv were:

- Who takes responsibility for website maintenance (i.e., security, software, hardware, plug-ins, resolving problems)? [2]

P. Smith (✉)
University of Florida, Gainesville, FL, USA
e-mail: plato.smith@ufl.edu

© The Author(s), under exclusive license to Springer Nature Switzerland AG 2023
M. R. Dreker, K. J. Downey (eds.), *Building Your Academic Research Digital Identity*, https://doi.org/10.1007/978-3-031-50317-7_7

- How are the costs of the website supported?
- What happens if the server or the software need upgrading? Who conducts the upgrade? Who pays the bill?
- Who takes responsibility for the content and updating the website? [3]

Although the post is related to sustainability of research project websites, the questions are imperative for developing and maintaining your personal academic identity website, particularly domain, software, and updates. Within the scope of this book chapter, some added measures to establish your academic digital identity include (a) embrace open access and open science, (b) develop an online personal website of your academic research career, (c) open access information—sharing your academic research and identifying collaborators, and (d) professional organizations followed by an ORCID iD quality control use case example as added measures to establish your digital identity.

Embrace Open Access and Open Science

What Is Open Access?

Open access can be defined as "there are no financial, legal or technical barriers to accessing [academic information such as publications and data]—that is to say when anyone can read, download, copy, distribute, print, search for and search within the information, or use [academic information] in education or in any way other within the legal agreements" [4]. The Berlin Declaration on Open Access to Knowledge in the Sciences and Humanities in 2003, is one the milestones of the Open Access (OA) movement supporting the transition to the electronic open access paradigm [5]. "Open access literature is digital, online, free of charge, and free of most copyright and licensing restrictions" [6]. Organizations, researchers, and librarians can embrace open access include supporting the open access by:

- Encourage researchers and recipients of grant funded research to publish their work according to the principles of the open access paradigm and data management and sharing requirements of funding agencies.
- Encourage the holders of cultural heritage and owners of academic information and research data to support open access by making publications and data freely available online.
- Develop resources to evaluate open access contributions and online journals to maintain the standards of quality assurance and good scientific practice.
- Advocating that open access publications be recognized in promotion and tenure evaluation.
- Advocate the intrinsic merit of contributions to open access infrastructure by software tool development, content provision, metadata creation, data curation, or the publication of individual articles [5].

The Scholarly Publishing and Academic Resources Coalition (SPARC) defines open access as "the free, immediate, online availability of research articles coupled with the rights to use these articles fully in the digital environment" [7].

Within the USA, "federal public access policy has been guided by the *Memorandum on Increasing Access to the Results of Federally Funded Research"* (2013 Memorandum) [8, 9]. The 2022 White House Office of Science and Technology Policy (OSTP) Memorandum states that "all peer-reviewed scholarly publications, authored or coauthored, by individuals or institutions resulting from federally funded research are made freely available and publicly accessible by default in agency-designated [data] repositories without any embargo of delay after publications" [9]. Data repositories can be domain-specific or generalist. "Domain-specific repositories are typically limited to data of a certain type or related to a certain discipline" [1]

In 2023 the OSTP announced new actions to advance open and equitable research through new grant funding, improvements in research infrastructure, and expanded public engagement opportunities [10]. OSTP, in efforts to advance open science policy across the federal government, is launching *Year of Open Science* throughout 2023 which includes providing access to the results of the nation's taxpayer-supported research [10]. Four key benefits of *open science* include: Citizen science initiatives and engagement; Lifesaving access to medical and scientific information; Democratization of the scientific process; and Increased Earth observation accessibility [11, 12].

What Is Open Science?

"Open science as such is not a new concept, and many terms have been used to refer to the transformation of scientific practices, such as Science 2.0 [13]. Multiple approaches that exist to the transformation to open science are all rooted in the tradition of openness of science. The European Commission started using the term "open science" as a result of the public consultation on Science 2.0 Science in Transition in 2014 (European Commission, 2015)" [12].

One Major Barrier to Open Access

One of the major barriers to open access is the financial costs associated with OA publishing. Recently I opted not to provide OA to an accepted peer-reviewed article, in a high-quality journal, due to OA article processing charges (APC) of $5000. An interesting opinion posted in Research Professional News in September 2022 stated that APC should reflect local economies and not promote inequity of the OA publishing financial model [14].

Example Solutions to Equitable Access

Sustainable and equitable business models that offer a wide range of benefits to researchers, libraries, and the community at large [13] are necessary to support open access. ScienceOpen Preprints offers a wide range of peer-review tools with no charge for preprint publication [15].

Open Access Committee at the University of Florida

In 2023 the University of Florida, George A. Smathers Libraries, Open Access Committee provided an update at the Library Town Hall meeting. The agenda included an Introduction, OA Initiatives, OA Evaluation Rubric, What's Next, and Share your feedback components. The section on article processing charges (APC) defined some key components of APC as:

- Used by some publishers or journals in lieu of subscription fees to support OA articles;
- Usually paid by authors, author institution, or funders;
- Some publishers offer agreements/contracts in which subscription costs reduce or eliminate APCs for authors (e.g., Articles published by Cambridge University Press will be available via Open Access with no additional charges to the library of UF authors) [16].

The George A. Smathers Library developed a very useful Open Access: UF Invests in OA: Memberships & Discounts library guide [17] which provides information on OA publishing models from Memberships (e.g., BioMed Central), Read & Publish (e.g., Cambridge University Press), Subscribe to Open (e.g., Annual Reviews), Collective Funding (e.g., SCOAP3), Library Publishing, and OA at UF status.

Develop an Online Personal Website of Your Academic Career

The author developed a personal website of his academic research career while completing his dissertation at Florida State University (FSU) School of Information in 2013 (see Fig. 7.1). The website includes name, current position, rank, and affiliation in the top heading of the website. The several headings of academic career include Research, Scholarly Works, Awards, Teaching, Service, and Curriculum Vitae.

The annual cost for web hosting in 2013 was $96.00. In 2021, the cost for a 2-year renewal was $203.28. The author added secure socket layer (SSL) to the domain site in 2022. The annual cost for SSL for the domain site is $25.00 which

7 Additional Measures to Establish Your Digital Identity

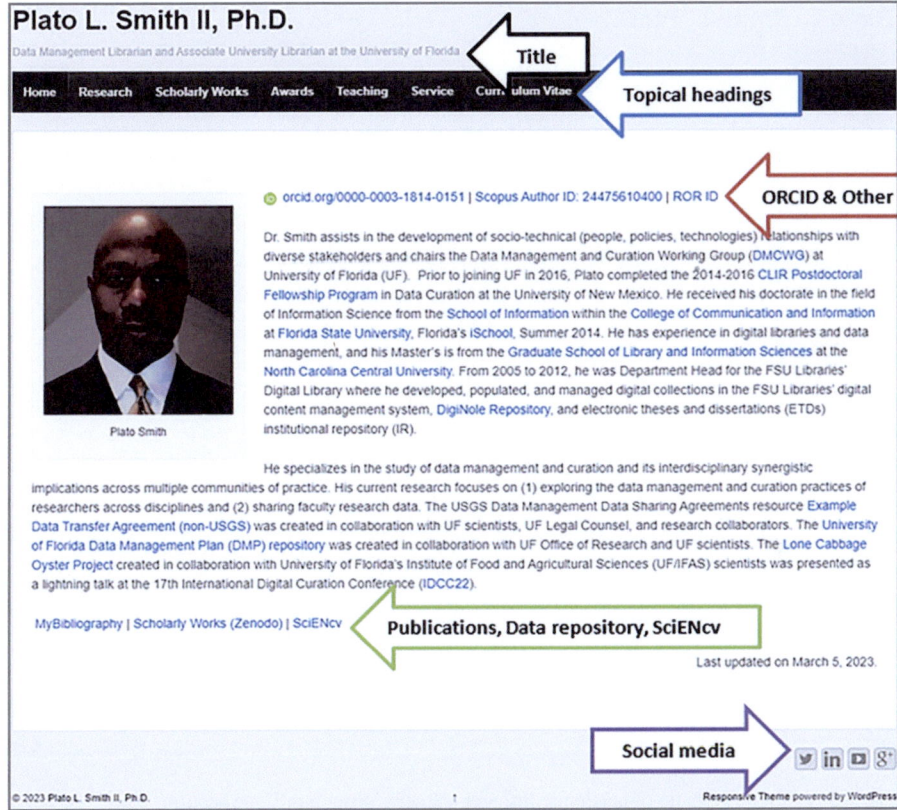

Fig. 7.1 Author's personal website of academic research career: https://platosmith.com/

allows you to have access to a website interface, control panel interface, and arxive support portal.

The Home page of his personal website illustrates an academic research digital identity. Figure 7.2 of the author's personal website titled Curriculum Vitae includes links to CV in PDF format, an ORCID profile, SciENcv, and Scopus Author ID. Leadership accomplishments, committee appointments, and the outputs can be listed here.

Where Do You Start in the Development of Your Personal Academic Research Website?

If you already have a personal website, then review it for necessary updates such as including other IDs. If you do not have a personal academic website like in Fig. 7.1, then start a personal website development plan for the aggregation and preservation of your academic career.

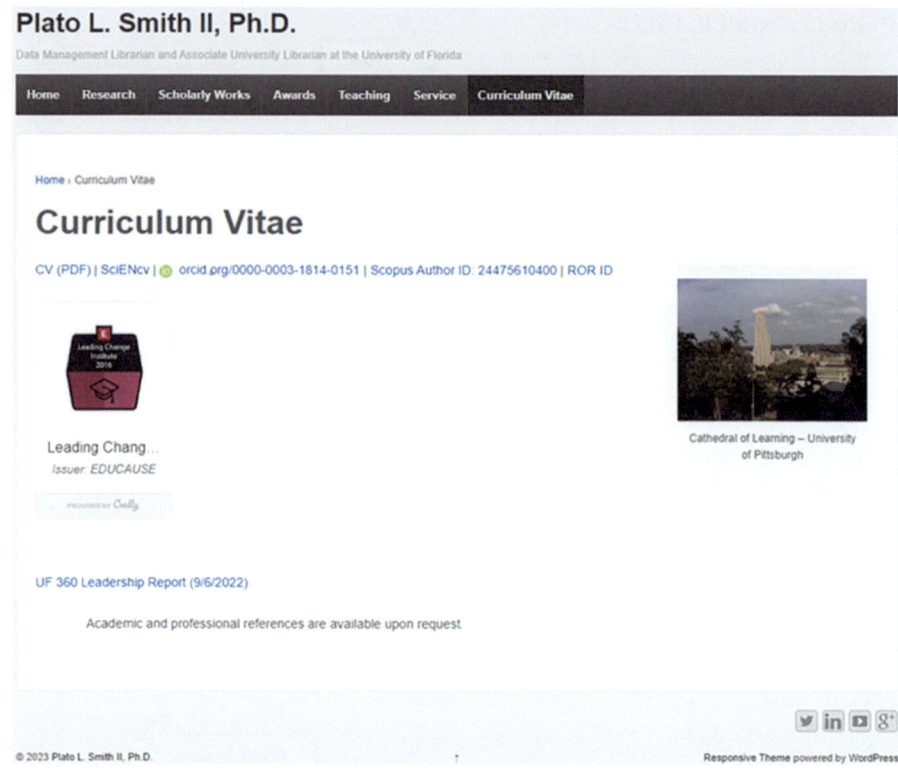

Fig. 7.2 Author's website of academic research career Curriculum Vitae section

Below Are Plans for Developing and Preserving Your Personal Academic Website

1. Make the committed decision to develop a personal website of academic/professional career.
2. Identify an exemplar model of an academic research career website you want to emulate.
3. Research current web hosting solutions.
4. Select the web hosting solution that best meets your current and future needs.
5. Decide on the primary use of a website to develop continuity in the progression of your academic career.
6. Prepare to budget for at least 10 years.
7. Decide on required software features options.
8. Install WordPress.
9. Select a theme.
10. Decide on plug-ins.
11. Develop the home page and topical heading categories.

7 Additional Measures to Establish Your Digital Identity

12. Prior experience working in Linux/Windows environment and web development are helpful.
13. Learn to code in HTML.
14. Read University of Kent Library and IT News How to Archive your website: https://blogs.kent.ac.uk/isnews/how-to-archive-your-website/
15. Review established website archiving online applications: The Internet Archive (https://archive.org/); UK Web Archive (https://www.webarchive.org.uk/en/ukwa/); WebCite (https://webcitation.org/); Mirrorweb (https://www.mirrorweb.com/).

Tools Used to Maintain a Digital Identity Throughout Your Academic Career

Developing, maintaining, and sustaining your digital identity requires active academic career lifecycle management. This includes but is not limited to checking, monitoring, tracking, and updating your various author profiles that make up your academic digital identity. You may have more than one academic digital identity such as Scopus Author ID and Web of Science Clarivate ResearcherID (see Chap. 5).

Your ORCID iD is a digital identity aggregator and integrator for including other ids as part of your ORCID profile. Your academic digital identity is a one-to-many relationship across platforms, publishers, and vendors. For example, the author's digital identity includes ORCID with funding award data from UF Integrated Research Support Tool (UFIRST) and Scopus Author ID to name a few (Fig. 7.3).

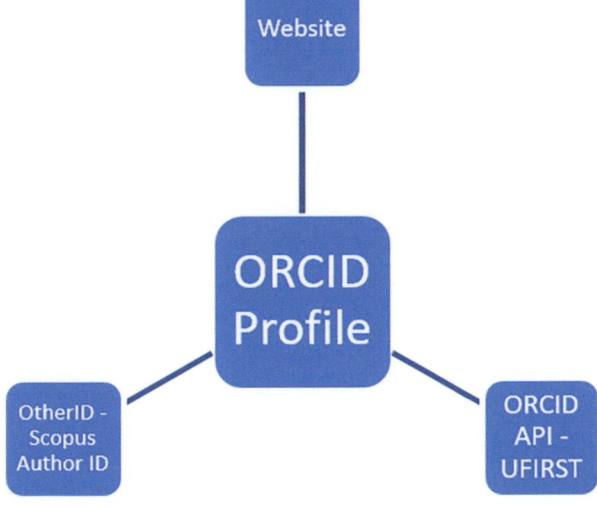

Fig. 7.3 Example of digital identity ORCID linked to Scopus Author ID and UFIRST (UF Integrated Research Support Tool) for proposal and award management at UF

Figure 7.3 illustrates how the author's academic identity is developed through ORCID which includes links to academic and professional websites, other identifiers such as Scopus Author ID.

Open Access Information: Share Your Data and Identifying Collaborators

One of the best recommendations for added measures to establish your digital identity is to contribute to a data repository that accepts publications, posters, presentations, datasets, images, video/audio, software, lessons, physical objects, and workflows. One of the many repositories available is Zenodo, https://zenodo.org, a general data repository powered by CERN Data Center and the invenio digital library framework, https://inveniosoftware.org/, for deposits of data.

Zenodo is free and has many features that can make your research findable, accessible, interoperable, reusable (FAIR). You can sign-in Zenodo using ORCID or GitHub credentials. You can archive GitHub code and software in Zenodo. The author developed the Scholarly Works community in 2016 (see Fig. 7.4) to store, share, and preserve select professional work to include on a website. You can create your own community in Zenodo to begin archiving and sharing your work. In 2019, graduate students at the University of Tennessee Knoxville School of Information Sciences [19] used Zenodo to store and share collaborative group projects (Fig. 7.5).

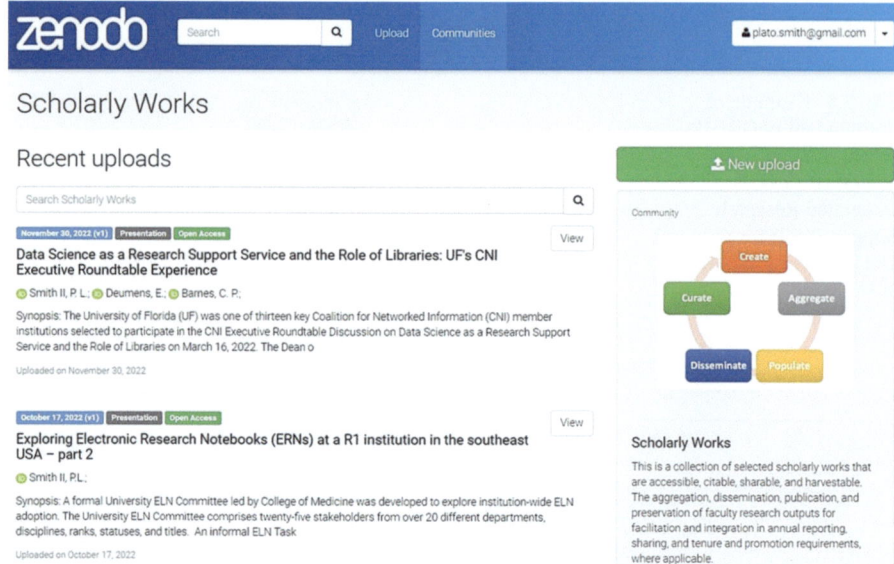

Fig. 7.4 Author's Scholarly Works [18] data repository in Zenodo linked from personal website

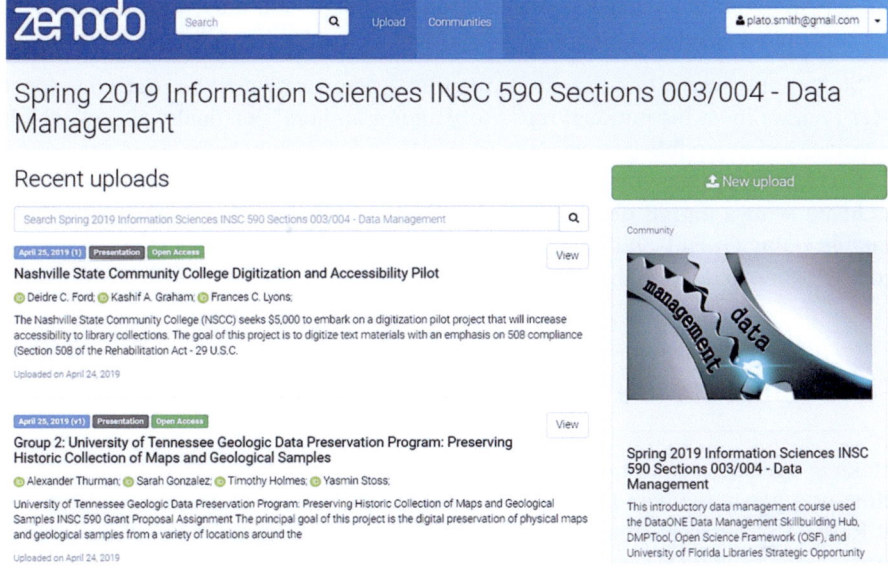

Fig. 7.5 Spring 2019 Information Sciences INSC 590 students' group projects in a data repository [19]

Promote Your Research to Increase Your Digital Identity

There are numerous added measures to establish your digital identity. According to Tennant [20], the top two key categories for increasing your digital identity are networking and maintaining your digital identity and sharing your research to enhance impact of your research. Tennant also provides a non-exhaustive top ten list of suggestions to increase your digital identity.

1. Place preprint/postreview articles on your institutional webpage or repository (e.g., Zenodo).
2. Place articles in an appropriate subject repository (e.g., arXiv, BiorXiv, SocArXiv, engXiv).
3. Inform interested users on social media platforms. Choose appropriate #hashtags or keywords to increase discoverability of your work (see Chap. 8).
4. Post links to articles on social media and any relevant groups, as well as academic networking sites, LinkedIn and Google+ profiles.
5. Save articles to your reference library and promote in the academic network of reference manager sites such as Mendeley or Zotero.
6. Share your research data and code (e.g., Figshare, Zenodo, GitHub).
7. Inform professional societies, news outlets, and bloggers in your field.
8. Create a Google Scholar profile and track citations.
9. Add articles to your ORCID account.

10. Update your ScienceOpen profile through ORCID and track your article-level and author-level metrics for all your research articles (see Chap. 6) [20].

Some publishers allow deposit of preprints (prepeer review) or postprints (post peer-review) in an institutional repository and/or authors' personal websites which is articulated in a publishers agreement.

Code, scripts, and software developed in GitHub repositories can be released and archived with a digital object identifier (DOI) in Zenodo. The Make Your Code Citable Using GitHub and Zenodo: A How-to Guide is a good reference on sharing your data and code to in increase your citations [21].

Store Your Data in a Research Data Repository

Funding agencies request depositing data in a data repository relevant to the discipline or a generalist data repository if domain-specific not available. The Registry of Research Data Repositories (re3data) is a resource to search for and discover data repositories to share research (See https://www.re3data.org/).

There are many repositories available within the National Institutes of Health (NIH) including the NIH Common Data Element (CDE) Repository, NIH Data Sharing Repositories, and the NIH Data Sharing Policies [22]. The NIH Data Sharing Repositories include Domain-Specific, and Generalist Repositories. The Generalist Repositories include: Figshare, Mendeley Data, Open Science Framework, and Zenodo.

Present Your Research at Conferences

Conference presentations are a valuable way of establishing your digital identity. There are a multitude of different conference platforms and as a presenter you want to take advantage of all these features to promote your research among your colleagues. You should take advantage of all the networking features that these online platforms offer. Hybrid and online conference presentations are ideal for promoting your academic research and digital identities.

Use Internal Organizational Tools

You can use internal organization tools such as blogs, departmental websites, faculty newsletters, media, and professional organizations to promote your digital identity. Developing collaborations with the administrators of the internal organization tools are crucial to the success of levering these tools to establish your digital identity. Figure 7.6 illustrates an internal organizational tool via blog spotlight titled *"Learn About a Lecturer."*

It will be your responsibility to discover any spotlights posted about you or your work. You may not have notifications set up, so it is recommended to check your internal resources. You can screen capture, link, and/or archive related works to develop your digital identity.

At the University of Florida, UF Apps is available to faculty. UF Apps provides access to software applications from any computer device-laptops, tablets, desktops, and smartphones [24]. Collaborations and partnerships with other campuses through advisory, committee, and working groups can enable awareness of internal organizational tools that can support development of your digital identity.

> After years of chairing the Data Management and Curation Working Group, the Director of Information Technology Research Computing shared that the agenda of a Faculty Senate IT meeting included electronic research notebook (ERN). After sending a brief ERN draft to the chair of the Faculty Senate IT Committee, the author was invited to give a brief update on ERN at the Faculty Senate IT meeting in October 17, 2022 resulting in the presentation posted to an internal organization website https://fora.aa.ufl.edu/FacultySenate/Pages/UniversityInformationTechnologyCommittee/AgendaMinutes2022-2023 (Electronic Research Notebooks).

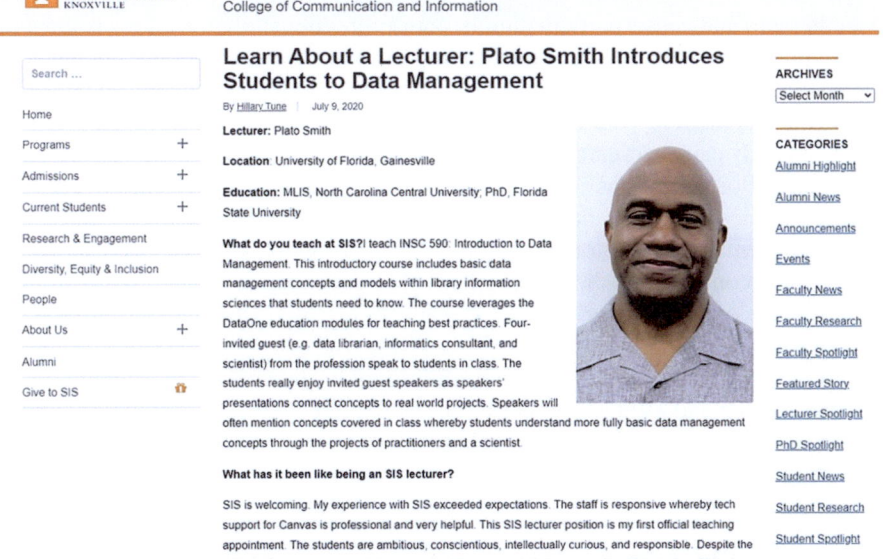

Fig. 7.6 University of Tennessee Knoxville School of Information Sciences spotlight Learn about a Lecturer (July 9, 2020) [23]

Another example of an internal organization tool is the University of Westminster blog titled "How sustainable is your research project website?" [25]. The blog details information related to institutional support for the development, planning, and sustainability of a research project website. The information provided on the blog can be adapted in the development of your personal academic career website.

Below are some institutional support websites that offer guidance on archiving and preserving your personal and project information.

- University of Kent—Research websites at Kent: https://www.kent.ac.uk/guides/research-websites-at-kent/after-your-project

    – University of Kent—Library and IT News: How to Archive your Website: https://blogs.kent.ac.uk/isnews/how-to-archive-your-website/

- University of Westminster: https://blog.westminster.ac.uk/researchoffice/how-sustainable-is-your-research-project-website/

The internal organization departmental website is another example of added measure to establish your digital identity. University of Florida's Academic Research Consulting & Services (ARCS) [26] department has a website that includes a "Featured Stories" column. Authored blogs and profile highlights can cultivate your digital identity.

Professional Organizations

Membership and active participation in your professional organizations is ideal for developing your networks that lead to opportunities for professional connections. Local, regional, national, and international societies and organizations all play roles in the development of your academic career.

As an early career researcher or academician, participation in local and statewide professional organizations is paramount. Getting involved in committee activities like conference planning, and being added to their listserv are useful ways to become an active member in these organizations. Participation in these professional organizations will contribute to the development of your academic career. Your institution may require or recommend outside organization participation for promotion and tenure purposes.

Membership in professional organizations will introduce key stakeholders within your discipline and establish important networking connections for future collaborations as well as the continuing development of your academic research career.

Recommendations

Recommendations include developing a personal academic/professional website of your career online. If your profile and research are distributed across multiple platforms, or with multiple vendors, or websites, then begin planning how to combine your data into a system in which you manage and control. Developing and professional website is best practice to store and manage this information. Review website archiving solutions as backup to your current or DIY website system. Before establishing your personal website there are three things you may want to explore:

1. **When Planning Your Personal Academic Website**
   - Review your organizational policies on having a personal website.
   - Make sure to add a professional headshot.
   - Review web hosting platforms.
   - Become familiar with the platform interface.
   - Understand the costs associated with establishing a website.
   - Understand there will be a time commitment in keeping your website current if you are planning on having a blog or column.
   - Become familiar with copyright policies.

2. **Updating and Associating Your Website with Other Digital Platforms**
   - Tying your website with your established digital profiles such as ORCID, Researcher ID, and Scopus ID.
   - Update your website with recent publications, presentations, talks, posters, abstracts, and other academic activities.
   - Make sure to list out your professional organizations and your service within the professional community.
   - Remove older or outdated information on your website.
   - Keep an updated academic calendar and record on your website which will allow colleagues to network with you at upcoming events.
   - Make sure to list out any current or ongoing research such as grants.

3. **Archiving—Your Website Should be Preserved for a Variety of Reasons:**
   - Be familiar with the tools needed to backup and archive your personal website.
   - The funder may require the website to be preserved for a given period.
   - The data and information on the website may still be useful and relevant to other researchers or users going forward and/or the purposes of research integrity [3].
   - Your organization may want to preserve your website in its data repository for historical reasons upon your retirement.
   - Make sure to place a disclaimer stating that your content is no longer being updated [3].

Conclusion

Develop a solid foundational academic or professional website on which to add, link, and promote your career. Using researcher profile platforms such as ORCID, Scopus Author ID, and SciENcv require management for quality control of information from other products in which your author profile data is shared.

Secure your ORCID iD account with two-factor authentication [27]. My NCBI SciENcv requires quality control monitoring of harvested information from ORCID which imports author research works from publishers (e.g., Scopus). Since the NSF will mandate SciENcv for biographical sketch in 2024, your ORCID and digital identity are important to your academic research career online.

In addition to maintaining a current, quality controlled ORCID iD, authors can share institution affiliation with Research Organization Registry (ROR) IDs. ROR is a community-supported open infrastructure that is driven by organizations and individuals from all over the world, and it includes persistent IDs and metadata for over 102,000 organizations" [28]. The National Institute of Standards and Technology (NIST) provides digital identity guidelines for federal agencies [29].

References

1. National Science Foundation. NSF-approved formats for the biographical sketch. 2023. https://new.nsf.gov/funding/senior-personnel-documents#biographical-sketch-0bd. Accessed 3 Jan 2024.
2. Schutt RK. Investigating the social world. 5th ed. Thousand Oaks: Sage; 2006.
3. Thomas M. How does your institution support websites beyond project life? 2023. https://tinyurl.com/2zeysumh. Accessed 21 Feb 2023.
4. Suber P. What is open access? https://tinyurl.com/ydgogxlu. Accessed 21 Feb 2023.
5. Max-Planck-Gesellschaft. Berlin declaration on Open Access to knowledge in the sciences and humanities. 2003. https://tinyurl.com/k8xdh7e. Accessed 21 Feb 2023.
6. Smith PL. Where IR you? Using "open access" to extend the reach and richness of faculty research within a university. OCLC Syst Serv. 2008;24:174–84.
7. SPARC. Open Access. 2023. https://tinyurl.com/yjgvlqje. Accessed 21 Feb 2023.
8. Holdren JP. Office of science and Technology Policy Memorandum for the Heads of Executive Departments and Agencies. 2013. https://tinyurl.com/ro97hwa. Accessed 21 Feb 2023.
9. Nelson A. Office of Science and Technology Policy (OSTP) Memorandum for the Heads of Executive Departments and Agencies. 2022. https://tinyurl.com/2ls2mt9v. Accessed 21 Feb 2023.
10. The White House Office of Science and Technology Policy. FACT SHEET: Biden-Harris administration announces new actions to advance open and equitable research. 2023. https://tinyurl.com/2ez4xh3u. Accessed 22 Feb 2023.
11. NASA. For researchers. Why do Open Science? 2023. https://tinyurl.com/2lfxgzvt. Accessed 22 Feb 2023.
12. Burgelman JC, Pascu C, Szkuta K, Von Schomberg R, Karalopoulos A, Repanas K, Schouppe M. Open Science, Open Data, and Open Scholarship: European policies to make science fit for the twenty-first century. Front Big Data. 2019;2:1–6.
13. Journal of City Climate Policy and Economy. Subscribe to Open. 2023. https://jccpe.utpjournals.press/journal/jccpe. Accessed 3 Mar 2023.
14. Osman F, Rooryck J. A fair pricing model for open access. 2022. https://tinyurl.com/2frtumw7. Accessed 21 Feb 2023.
15. ScienceOPEN. 2023. https://www.scienceopen.com/. Accessed 3 Mar 2023.
16. Gallagher E, Ye H. Open Access Committee. Presented at the George A. Smathers Libraries at the University of Florida Town Hall. Virtual. 2023.

17. UF George A. Smathers Libraries. Open access: UF invests in OA: memberships & discounts. 2023. https://guides.uflib.ufl.edu/openaccess/ufinvests. Accessed 22 Feb 2023.
18. Thomas M. How does your institution support websites beyond project life? 2023. https://tinyurl.com/2f626rll. Accessed 1 Mar 2023.
19. Smith PL II. Spring 2019 information sciences INSC 590 sections 003/004: data management. 2019. https://tinyurl.com/rs94txd. Accessed 24 Feb 2023.
20. Tennant J. Promoting your articles to increase your digital identity and research impact. scienceopen.com. 2017. https://tinyurl.com/2mao2f3m. Accessed 3 Mar 2023.
21. Open Science MOOC. Make your code citable using GitHub and Zenodo: a how-to guide. 2018. https://genr.eu/wp/cite/. Accessed 6 Mar 2023.
22. NIH NLM. Trans-NIH Biomedical Informatics Coordinating Committee (BMIC). 2022. https://www.nlm.nih.gov/NIHbmic/index.html. Accessed 25 Feb 2023.
23. University of Tennessee Knoxville School of Information Sciences. Learn about a lecturer: Plato Smith introduces students to data management. 2020. https://tinyurl.com/2zdeaho2. Accessed 22 Feb 2023.
24. UF IT. Apps. 2023. https://info.apps.ufl.edu/. Accessed 3 Jan 2024.
25. Ranger H. How sustainable is your research project website? 2022. https://tinyurl.com/2pnuuwvn. Accessed 22 Feb 2023.
26. UF George A. Smathers Libraries. Academic Research Consulting & Services. Featured stories. https://arcs.uflib.ufl.edu/stories/. Accessed 23 Feb 2023.
27. ORCID. Secure your account with two-factor authentication. 2022. https://tinyurl.com/2qwwpqxl. Accessed 28 Feb 2023.
28. ROR. What is ROR? 2023. https://ror.org/about/. Accessed 3 Mar 2023.
29. Grassi PA, Garcia ME, Fenton JL. National Institute of Standards and Technology (NIST), NIST Special Publication 800-63 Revision 3, digital identity guidelines. 2017. https://pages.nist.gov/800-63-3/sp800-63-3.html. Accessed 3 Jan 2024.
30. Jasini K. Shared information about an author's institutional affiliation: Introducing ROR IDs. 2023. https://tinyurl.com/2ej2judy. Accessed 3 Mar 2023.

Chapter 8
Building Your Digital Presence on Social Media

Matthew Bridgeman

Introduction

How many times have you heard a speaker online or at a conference and looked them up online? Do they have a social media account? What happens when they don't have one, or it is poorly done, and you are not quite sure the profile is the speaker? What was your impression? Now imagine the inverse, that is someone looking for you after hearing you talk. What type of image do you want them to see? What will it say?

Today we meet people, formally or informally, online and we have to ask ourselves "what are they seeing," or rather "who are they seeing?" First impressions matter and they tend to be made the instant they see you or your online presence. Thankfully they skew positive but tend to be plagued with stereotypes [1].

It is estimated that 72% of the people in the world have some social media presence. In the short time it has been around it quickly became a way to connect with like-minded people [2].

The goals of this chapter are to help select the best platform and provide strategies to build an effective presence on that platform. There are hundreds of platforms available, and it would be impossible to list them all. We will be discussing a sample of the most popular platforms and provide guidance on how to effectively use them to promote your scholarly presence. This approach will provide you with a variety of skills you can utilize across multiple platforms.

Social media is currently the most direct way to engage in scholarly discussion, and its importance seems to be only growing [3]. It is important to consider how you establish yourself and how to use the tools to your advantage. Afterall, anything we post can be cited. As default there are no limits or qualifications to participate in social media, so it is important to establish yourself by building a unique

M. Bridgeman (✉)
Rutgers University, New Brunswick, NJ, USA
e-mail: mcb226@libraries.rutgers.edu

© The Author(s), under exclusive license to Springer Nature Switzerland AG 2023
M. R. Dreker, K. J. Downey (eds.), *Building Your Academic Research Digital Identity*, https://doi.org/10.1007/978-3-031-50317-7_8

enough image to stand out as a credible presence. In addition, social media may be an effective way to reach out to new researchers as they may not have the benefit of a library system and they would rely on google for primary articles farming [4]. While at one point it may seem to have been enough to publish to become known as a scholar, it seems to be increasingly true that you must have a social media presence to be more involved in academic discourse [5].

Social Media Platforms

Social media is a collection of highly connected and highly visible software designed to create connections. Chances are you are already participating in one of the several platforms available: Instagram, LinkedIn, Facebook, Twitter (X), etc.

There are a few "scholar centric" platforms such as ResearchGate and Academia. edu. When approaching these platforms, it is important to keep in mind what they are: big data tools. They use the data you provide in profiles, interactions, posts, connections, and clicks to function. Understanding how they use data can be an invaluable skill that will help you build an effective online presence.

The information below highlights the major functions and features of several social media platforms. This will provide you with a foundation for building your profile by giving you the basics on how these platforms work. Even if a platform is not listed you can apply the same analytic approach by reviewing the function and overview of the features before building your profile.

Building a Digital Profile on Social Media

Social media platforms require you to create an account to begin using their features. Most of the time these are free, though several have premium features that come with a fee. These accounts are based on your profile. A profile is the foundational information you provide including name, biographical information, interests, employment history, etc. To properly build your presence as a scholar on social media, you must have an appropriate profile. Not only is it the primary source of information other accounts can see, but the information provided will impact how the platform interacts with you. This segment will cover profile design and tips to help you develop an effective scholarly presence.

In his 2021 article, Prabhu outlines three guiding principles for approaching social media that focuses on scholarship:

1. Identify your personal goals.
2. Identify preferred media format, blogs, videos, podcasts.
3. Identify "influencers" or experts in your field [5].

Take these three principles into account when building a profile and later curating your presence.

What are your goals for using social media? As a scholar it could be building relationships for future collaboration, discussing, and debating ideas, or simply networking with colleagues. Once you identify your goals it will make selecting the best platform easy then you can begin searching for other "influencers," or people in the same field of ones you find interesting.

The data you enter in your profile will affect the information the platform will push to you including "people you may know" and news in your profession. It will also affect where you may appear in suggested areas. If you include your complete job history, the more recent institution will get the most attention. Your profile will be the starting point before you can start influencing the data processes.

General Tips for Establishing a Digital Profile on Social Media

Create a Dedicated Email Account for Social Media

One caveat with any social media account is their remarkable ability to create email clutter. Although some email services, such as Gmail, can organize your emails into categories, it is still recommended to create a social media only account. Not only will it help organize the flow of email, but it will also improve your mental health by creating a barrier between social media and everything else. With that said, do not use your work email for social media.

Profile Pictures

According to LinkedIn's research, an account with a profile picture is 14 times more likely to have someone interact with it. This will be the first impression a user sees before they read the rest of your profile. When your profile is accessed, the corresponding banner image will appear at the top of your profile. This can work together to establish an impressive presence. This combination of images is a template which can be utilized across all platforms since many have the same design of a small circle profile picture with a large banner in the background [6].

LinkedIn provides some tips for profile pictures:

- Be the only person in the profile picture.
- Your face should be most of the image.
- Use a high-resolution image.
- No "selfies."

- The background should be clean.
- Take the photograph outside or with a solid background.

Banner Images

Banner images are long rectangular images that are both for the heading of your profile and the background. Including a banner image is beneficial and you have slightly more flexibility with the banner. It can be a color or a landscape, but it can't be messy.

Keep the banner image simple. A crowded banner can be distracting to the viewer. If possible, make it work related. Most institutions will have a visual identity page you can use.

LinkedIn

LinkedIn was founded in 2003, making it the oldest platform discussed in this chapter. In 2015, it acquired the learning service lynda.com which offers continuing education online. It was an independent entity until it was bought by Microsoft in 2016. It bills itself as the world's largest professional network with over 850 million members worldwide. Its emphasis on professional connections makes this the ideal platform for connecting with other scholars to discuss research. Odds are this may also be the first place someone will look for information on you.

LinkedIn Functions

The structure of LinkedIn is based on the six degrees of separation. It is the idea that all people are six or fewer connections away from each other. There is some debate on the truth of this, but it is compelling, nonetheless.

Though instead of six, LinkedIn has three degrees and each degree has differing levels of capabilities related to your profile. These degrees of connection will be labeled on the profile in the top right corner. You will be visible to all degrees, but your level of interaction varies with each level. A profile not within the 3 degrees is called "out-of-network" and they won't appear in your feed, but you can still search for them [7].

First-Degree Connections

First-degree connections are formed when two profiles accept invitations for a connection. The analogy would be your coworker you work with and know. You can directly message them and communicate.

Second-Degree Connections

Second-degree connections are formed when someone becomes a first-degree connection with one of your first-degree connections, but they are not connected to you. You cannot message them because you are not linked through an invite yet. Think of them as a friend of a coworker you have not met yet.

Third Degree Connections

Third degree connections are when someone accepts and invites from a second-degree connection. You cannot interact with them, and you can't see their full name.

Followers

Followers can see posts but are not connected in any of the three degrees. You can have followers and you can follow other profiles [7].

LinkedIn Features

Profile Views

One feature that is unique to LinkedIn is the ability to see who viewed your profile. The reach of the feature is limited by your level of membership. At the basic level you can see only your close connections, while a premium subscription allows you to see all who reviewed your profile. You can only see people who have viewed your profile in the past 90 days.

Multimedia Capabilities

LinkedIn supports video and presentation software. If you have a recorded presentation you are proud of you can upload it for people to view. They also have the option to upload PowerPoints and images you would like to share with other scholars.

Interest Groups

A LinkedIn group is a subject specific page where people with shared interests can post and have discussions with each other. You do not need to share a connection with any of the members, but it may help if you are familiar with people in the group. If a group does not exist, you are free to create one [8].

Posts

You can write posts that pop up under your profile and will be shared with your connections and followers. There is a 3000-character limit on posts. You can include tags, hashtags, and links. Tags use the @ symbol to link profiles to your post and hashtags use the # symbol to link your posts to subjects thereby making it more discoverable. You can also comment or interact with any post regardless of connection. You may include images, videos, documents, and even prepare a short article.

Premium Subscriptions

Premim subscriptions include LinkedIn learning, formerly lynda.com. It allows you to see people who have reviewed your profile regardless of degree relationship. The premium subscription is focused on job searches and business growth. It may be helpful if you are just starting or looking for a job, but not necessary for long term profile uses. It includes InMail credits which allows you to message someone you are not connected to.

LinkedIn Profile Tips

LinkedIn is based on connecting people through their profession. As a result, creating a profile is not dissimilar to filling out an online job application. Except you only need to do it once. You need to include your employment history, educational background, certifications, accomplishments, and more.

When building your profile, take your time with each step of the process so you can share only what you want to be shared. They may ask for your contact list to link you with contacts already in the platform. However, this had caused some controversy in the past. In June 2015, the company agreed to pay $13 million to settle a class action lawsuit resulting from sending multiple email invitations to users' contact lists [9]. The following segment is organized in the same manner as LinkedIn with core, recommended, and additional categories.

Basic Components of a LinkedIn Profile

The basic components include employment history, education and skills. It is essentially your Curriculum Vitae (CV). Be sure both are up to date. If it is in your CV, it should be in your profile including job experiences, education, and relevant skills. When you include a skills, it will need to be selected from a list. There are no limits on skills so include as many as are relevant to you and your scholarship.

Core

About You

You can begin your narrative here by telling a story about how you got started and where you are going. It should contain a summation of your current position and research interests. It has a 2600-character limit, which translates to roughly 500 words [10].
Recommended Structure

- Current Position information.
- Beginning of career and any interesting projects.
- Research areas and future goals.

Featured

The featured section of your profile is where you can highlight your accomplishments. You can upload posters, presentations, videos, links, and articles published in LinkedIn. There is a lot of flexibility in the content you can upload, but no pdfs.

Additional Information

The additional group includes publications, awards, and professional organizations. It would be beneficial to include that information. However, it does not need to be exhaustive. Include publication and presentations that highlight your strengths and your areas of research.

Audio for Name Pronunciation

You can include a 10-s clip to help with name pronunciation. In such a diverse field as academia, it may be helpful to provide a quick audio on how to pronounce your name.

LinkedIn is the most formal platform, meaning you focus on your professional connections and building a scholarly network. The suggested schedule for posting is about once a week. Some resources will say to post multiple times in a week which could be helpful but may be unsustainable in the long run.

It is a tool for promoting scholarship, not the scholarship itself. Social media has been studied to be addictive and you want to avoid it becoming a burden. When you do post make sure the posts are primarily related to your field or profession. That will maintain your presence in the field which will keep you in the feed of your various connection levels. These posts don't have to be long or in-depth, as long as they are consistent.

Building Your Connections

When you begin on LinkedIn it immediately begins building your connections and your feed based on the information you provided in your profile. This will include suggested connections from places you have worked, educational history, and places you have lived. If you have built a solid profile, it will be easy to begin creating that first level of connections that will reach out to the next two levels. Keep in mind that the second and third level connections may be people you do not know. However, individual profile connections are for people you have met, maybe at a conference or at a networking event.

Liking or Commenting

If you like or comment on a post from someone else, it will show up in your connections feed. This is a great way to promote scholarly discussion among colleagues. This will also teach the platform to share relevant scholarly content with you. For example, articles about institutions and research programs that are in your field. Search for topics and articles related to your field and begin liking, sharing and commenting on them. This will bring more relevant content to your feed and make you more visible in your field of interest. Also, it will increase the probability of those accounts commenting on your posts.

LinkedIn Posts

Posts are the best way to build your presence on LinkedIn. We have briefly touched on post frequency on LinkedIn, about once a week. The primary rationale is that posts often require more work than sharing a link or an interesting article. LinkedIn has a great deal of flexibility when coming to posts. They can be almost any length and include images, videos, and other files. Think of them as miniature articles that you are writing. Research has many stages, and you can keep people updated on your own scholarship while also creating mini articles. There are plenty of websites and blog posts that describe how to prepare the perfect post. When creating a post use no more than 5 hashtags [11].

LinkedIn allows a variety of post types and lengths from a few dozen characters to full length articles. The survey information provided by LinkedIn suggests either short posts, only a sentence or two, or a lengthy article of 1500 words. Anything in between does not receive as much engagement [11].

LinkedIn Groups

Groups are designated chat rooms where you can have a group discussion on a particular topic. You can join or create your own group. Odds are there is already a group for you, so making a new one is not recommended, at least not at the start. It is recommended to start searching for your local library association or organization. There are groups for every region of the Medical Library Association. Engaging with these groups is a great way to establish your presence to a large group of professionals.

ResearchGate

ResearchGate was founded in 2008 and it is the largest academic focused social media platform with over 20 million profiles. This platform is designed for sharing research and promoting scholarly discussion. You are free to upload pdfs of your articles for others to access. In a 2017 paper, which surveyed early career researchers, ResearchGate was mentioned the most as a resource for articles [4].

Since there is no copyright protection component of RG, it is possible to share materials that violate copyright [12]. In 2022, publishers Elsevier and the American Chemical Society filed a lawsuit based on individuals uploading copyrighted material. The result of the lawsuit says the platform is responsible for uploaded papers, but enforcement of any policy has not been established [13]. It is imperative you are familiar with the copyright status and sharing permissions on your publications before uploading them.

ResearchGate Functions

ResearchGate, as the name implies, is research focused and is designed around research topics and making connections. Unlike the other platforms discussed here, there are no recommended posts. It is entirely profile based, you only see the content you follow. This gives a user more control to curate the content they want to interact with. The platform gains revenue from advertising by using your profile information to create a targeted add [14].

ResearchGate Features

Question and Answer

Unlike most social media platforms, ResearchGate does not have a post feature, instead it has Question and Answer. Here members can post a question related to their research. You can add subject terms to the question to optimize searches. It can then be answered by any other member and shared on other social media platforms. In addition, it can show relevant research articles available within ResearchGate.

Uploading Articles to ResearchGate

You can upload articles that you published to ResearchGate. These articles can also be found using google, and is often a source of literature searching [4]. As we mentioned previously, this aspect has gotten the platform into legal trouble. As a result the future of this feature is uncertain.

RG Scores

The RG score is the proprietary metric used by ResearchGate. It is affected solely by your interactions within the platform. It takes into account the information your provide and the relationships you build with other profiles. The specifics on how this number is calculated is not shared by the platform. However, it should be approached as how effective your account is and not as a formal metric even then, it should not be the focus of your profile.

ResearchGate Profile

You have 500 characters to write your introduction. All your work and publication information is available. Use this space to provide an overview of your research and future directions. You are preparing an elevator pitch.

The Mignone Center for Career Services at Harvard University provides an excellent outline for an elevator pitch that can be adapted to writing an introduction.

- Who are you?
- What do you do?
- What's unique about you?
- Call to Action.
- Something Memorable (Optional) [15].

Question and Answer Posts

Utilizing the "Question and Answer" feature is the primary way of engaging other profiles in ResearchGate. It is also the best way to highlight your scholarly expertise while also getting you noticed by your peers.

Before you write a question, search to see if something similar was already asked. Length of an answer depends on the question. Though don't be afraid of providing a detailed response. When asking a question, be as clear as possible and try to keep the length short. If you find yourself writing a long question, see if it is possible to break it up into two or more smaller questions. If you have a question from an article, attach it as a reference.

RG Messages

This is the least effective but most direct form of communication in ResearchGate. Messaging other researchers is reserved for profiles in which you know the researcher, or you have a specific question about their scholarship.

RG Disciplines

You can include multiple disciplines from a drop-down menu. Information science is related to computer science. You may want to include your liaison area or subject specialization; however, it is not recommended. You can provide more accurate details in the Skills and Expertise segment.

Skills and Expertise

Select five skills and expertise from the menu. Highlight your profession and your strengths related to your research. They function the same as a hashtag in which too many will harm discoverability.

Research

Due to the current issues with copyright, it is not recommended to upload any articles. If it is open access, then you are free to upload the pdf. However, you should input all your publication citation information, which can include a link to the article. Input anything and everything you published from blog posts to peer-reviewed articles. If you have co-authors, let them know you are inputting the information in ResearchGate. The more work you store in RG, the larger presence you will have.

Twitter or X

Twitter or X, (Twitter was rebranded as X in July, 2023) was launched in 2006 and it went public in 2013. It then went private again in 2022. It has over 237 million active users. 25 to 34-year-olds are the primary users of Twitter. It describes itself as a microblogging platform where an individual can post short blurbs about anything.

Twitter Or X Function

Twitter is designed with a simple interface: a profile and a feed. The feed is an endless list of tweets from followers, recommended accounts, and advertisements. Their primary source of revenue is advertising, so they can be a bit heavy, especially if your account is not active. The information in your feed is based on the profiles you follow and create. If you are not active the feed will remain generic and filled with trending topics. Once you post a tweet it is available and searchable through the Twitter platform. Tweets cannot be searched outside the platform such as through Google, Bing, Duck Duck Go and other search engines. You can share a protected tweet that only your followers can see, however it does come with some caveats that are explained below.

@: The @ symbol links a profile to a tweet and instantly shows up in their account feed, and they will receive a notification.

#: Hashtags are used to assign terms to a tweet. This allows the tweet to appear when people search that hashtag. They are the equivalent of subject headings.

Recommendations on posting on Twitter:

- Tweet once or twice a day.
- Comment and like other tweets.
- Monday–Thursday between 1pm and 3pm has been shown to be an effective time to post [16].

Twitter or X Features

Followers

Followers are other Twitter profiles that find your content interesting and essentially subscribe to your account to include your tweets in their feed.

Tweets

The Primary form of interaction on Twitter. It has a 280-character limit (a Twitter Blue account allows users to post up to 10,000 characters per post). They can be deleted. Here you can expand the reach of your tweet by using hashtags and the @ symbol. You can also include images and share links to interesting articles.

Tweets are meant to be memorable and easy to read, so it is recommended to keep them fairly short with only one or two hashtags. This increases the chance of someone reading it while scrolling and engaging with the tweet.

You can use emojis but sparingly. A few will add color, but too many and it will affect the perceived reliability.

When attending events, conferences, or talks, always mention the speaker or event in the tweet. Everyone loves some recognition, especially if you find the content engaging [3, 17].

Protected Tweets

These are tweets that only your followers can see. You can even make past tweets protected, however if someone had included that tweet in their timeline before it became protected, it will remain visible [18].

Video Tweets

You can upload up to 2 min and 20 second videos to Twitter. This can be done by uploading a file or shooting the video in Twitter where you can edit the video. Videos play automatically as default, but you can change that in the settings.

Threads

Threads are a long chain of interconnected tweets. They can be a multipart tweet written by you as a way to exceed the character limit. They can also be a discussion on a single tweet in which you respond to comments.

Threads are not recommended, because they go against the microblogging ideal of Twitter. If you must post something that is longer than a tweet, use a high-resolution image of a text file such as a word document or google doc. This trick bypasses the character count and presents the text in a clean single tweet.

Polls

The poll feature allows you to set up a poll and receive real time feedback on a question. These polls allow a single question to be posted at a time. You can close the poll at any time and share the results with your followers.

Verified Accounts

These are accounts in which the profile has been established as genuine. This was done in an effort to fight imposter accounts and stem the spread of misinformation. In late 2022 an account could be verified through a paid subscription service called Twitter Blue. Though previously verified accounts remained as "legacy" accounts.

Twitter or X Profile Tips

Creating a Handle

The handle is your Twitter account name. It is like selecting a telephone number, there can't be duplicate accounts. Though you may find mimic handles that only change a few letters or include numbers to fake being a legitimate account. There are default handles Twitter will suggest, but it is best to create one that clearly identifies you and your interests. Take your time picking a handle. If possible, try for something short and easily read. Once you select one it is permanent, meaning you will never be able to change it without creating a new account.

Biography

The profile has a maximum of 160 characters, so there is not much room to tell your life story. Instead, you can include a favorite quote or outline your current area of research.

Website

If you have a website or another social media account, you can place a link here, but use a link shortener like bit.ly or tinyurl.com. You can also check if your institution has a proprietary link shortener.

Instagram

Instagram was launched in 2010 and it was acquired by Meta (formerly Facebook) in 2012. It is an image and video focused platform. It initially grew in popularity due to its image filter feature. They would give photographs some added color and depth. As it grew, more features were added including stores, video streams, reels, and even a shopping feature. The primary demographic on Instagram is 18 to 34 [19]. This would be a good platform for younger researchers. There are concerns over Instagram affecting mental health related to body image or unrealistic situations.

Instagram Function

Instagram is a visual platform where the primary content is images and videos. Profiles consist only of a profile image and a brief biography. You engage with other profiles through, follows, likes, comments, and time spent on viewing posts. These engagements then affect what you are shown. For example, if you spend time looking at anatomy sites and pictures, you will get suggested more of the same by the platform's algorithms.

Instagram Features

Images and Filters

You can post pictures you have taken or images you made. You can then apply image filters such as black and white, sepia toned, and dozens of others to add some extra flair to your posts.

Videos

Videos can be 3–60 seconds long with or without sound and appear in the same feed as images. They have the same functionality as images.

Reels

Introduced in 2020, reels are 15–30 seconds clips you can post in your reels section of your profile. These were introduced to compete with TikTok and have become a popular feature. Reels are the best way to engage with other profiles on Instagram. Since they are so popular some people have been posting exclusively to reels instead of their main image feed. The way reels are shared is through hashtags and behind the scenes algorithms. To enhance your scholarly presence, it is essential for you to post reels related exclusively to your research areas or profession.

Stories

Stories are posts that exist for 24 hours and exist in the stories feed, separate from the post feed. They are often used to highlight certain posts, activities, or tell a story through images such as your time at a conference. Stories are videos that last 24 hours before self-deleting. Their temporary nature means they can be less formal and not strictly focused on scholarship. They can be more fun. As their name suggests they are good for telling stories that take place over a period of time. Stories are especially effective during conferences or long projects because they can serve as updates and demonstrate progress. Stories can also be archived by the user by using the highlight feature. This feature allows other users to see your past stories that you have choosen to highlight and remain archived on your profile.

Instagram Profile

Instagram allows you to build a small profile which includes a biography, pronouns, name, and links.

Instagram Biography

Begin your biography with your current job title or profession. For example, Information and Education Librarian at Rutgers University. Then follow with one sentence summary on your research topic. You can also include something fun about yourself or your job. You can sacrifice grammar for brevity when preparing these bios, due to the 150-character limit.

Sample Biography:

Librarian at Robert Wood Johnson Health Sciences Library, NJ.
Specializes in open access education resources and drug information resources.

Links

This is the only place you can insert permanent links. The basic links to include are to your workplace, videos you have created, and interesting articles or publications you have written. Not only will this reinforce your presence, but it may also boost your impact factor. You can also promote links to studies you are conducting or webinars you have hosted.

Instagram Posts

Since the content of Instagram is primarily visual, you will need to curate your images to make them engaging and relevant to your scholarship. The library field has limited opportunities for images if you focus just on the buildings and stacks, even though they are some of the most iconic images associated with the profession. Instagram is best used when it features images of people at a conference or sharing images of your workspace. These images can be less formal to let your personality shine.

A recent research article on library Instagram's offers some useful analysis of content that is effective and used by libraries. They broke down posts into a fixed set of categories: Interacting, orienting, placemaking, and showcasing. Each of these categories can be used by a scholar as well. Interactive posts can be you asking the audience for a response, either through messaging or comment. Orienting posts show your place in a space. This can be your workplace, workstation, places you can visit nearby that are related to your work. Placemaking posts highlight the things that make you, you. These are images of how you represent your ideology and personality. They are the most enjoyable and probably the posts with the highest engagement [20].

Instagram Posts Tips

1. Posting between 11:00 am and 12:00 pm is the best time to maximize your reach [21].
2. Photographs should have high contrast to stand out from other posts. In other words, make sure there is some color [22].
3. Images with people in them get the most interaction. You can post images of your work place or update on the status of your scholarship. If you publish, post a celebration image and thank co-authors if you have them.
4. Hashtag limit: 5 is the recommended limit on hashtags, but you can use more or less if the post requires it. However, try to keep it within this range.

Video

Video is a little challenging for scholarly presence. Though think of Instagram videos as images but with depth. Use a video to highlight a single topic or detail you would like to share. For example, if you take a picture at a conference, use a video and show around the convention floor and highlight talks or topics you are interested in or participating in. Be sure to keep the videos less than 30 seconds long.

Facebook

In 2024, it is hard to imagine someone who has not heard of Facebook. Launched in 2004 it began as a university/college only platform. It is designed as a way to meet people online through shared interests. It has since grown into a multi-media and multifunctional platform that is involved in nearly every aspect of our lives from politics to shopping. Its primary demographic are individuals between the ages of 18 and 44, who compose 59.8% of users [23].

With over 2.9 billion users, it is the largest social media platform, and as of 2022 the second most visited website in the world. Since its growth, it acquired other platforms such as Instagram. Facebook is also the center of a multitude of controversies from misinformation, data and privacy violations, antitrust litigation and more. Like with any social media platform, it is best to approach this with some caution [24].

Facebook Functions

The foundation of Facebook's functions is your profile. The profile includes biographical information, interests, hobbies, and other personal details. Facebook uses this information to connect you with similar people, companies, and businesses. They also use this information to populate your feed also known as your timeline. Facebook's primary revenue source is advertising which is conducted through targeted ads. These ads are selected based on the information in your profile, the profiles you follow, and the content you interact with. The goal is to get you to engage with content. Like with other platforms, an inactive profile will become populated with almost exclusively ads or popular content [25].

Facebook Features

Facebook Profile

Your Facebook profile is your main account with several information categories in which you input information. It also acts as a hub of all your posts and stories uploaded files such as videos and images [26].

Many of the "profile tips" already discussed on other platforms will apply to Facebook, such as using the elevator pitch structure for your biography, and the guidelines for profile and banner images.

Facebook allows you to input more personal information than the other platforms such as birthday and location. You are under no obligation to provide that personal information if you are not comfortable. You may choose to focus solely on your scholarly identity such as education, work information, and scholarly pursuits.

The biggest challenge with Facebook is if you already have a long-standing personal profile. You cannot create a new profile just for scholarly content. It would be confusing to have duplicate accounts. Transforming your current profile from personal to professional would be a substantial undertaking. The best option would be to create an account on another platform.

Facebook Feed

The feed is an auto-generated and endless list of content that is affected by the information you provide in your profile, the profiles you follow, and the interactions you have with content.

Facebook Posts

Facebook posts are also called status updates where you can provide a couple sentences on anything. You can posts links, videos, and images. They have a 33,000-character limit, the largest of all platforms. Other people can comment or interact with your posts, unless you set them to private.

Facebook is less formal than LinkedIn, which means your posts don't have to be primarily work related. Here you can have more fun and allow more of your personality shine.

Facebook allows you to post links to websites and videos. This allows you to create posts with minimal effort. Only links or status updates can make your Facebook feed look monotonous and uninteresting. Providing a mix of links, videos, and short blurbs can be effective.

Below are some tips for posts that will keep your account interesting and promote engagement.

1. Post 3 or 4 times a week at the most.
2. Post interest articles, videos, or news items.
3. Comments are encouraged, especially if you find something interesting related to your field.

Facebook Groups

Facebook groups are private chat rooms focused on a shared interest. There are three types of groups. In public groups, anyone can read or post within the group. In private groups, only members can read or make posts. Secret groups, are unsearchable and available through invite only.

Groups are the best way to engage with a community. In fact, they are also one of the best ways to enhance your scholarly presence because they have a lot of weight in their algorithm. In other words, if you communicate in a Facebook group, your profile and posts will appear more prominently in relevant areas and vice versa.

It is not recommended to start your own group. They require a great deal of work to establish, and if your area of expertise is small it may not ever become fully realized. If you find a need for a community, or it grows out of another, then it may be feasible to create and maintain a new group.

Shared Features with Other Platforms

You may notice Facebook has some of the same features as Instagram such as reels and stories. That's because they are both owned by the parent company Meta. You can link both platforms and share posts between the two.

Other Social Media Platforms

There are countless social media platforms and some that may be of interest as demonstrated below. (Table 8.1).

Writing Your Narrative: Profile Upkeep and Curation.

When you create a profile, you lay the foundation for your digital identity. When you create content, you are telling your story. What narrative about yourself and your scholarship are you writing? Think of social media as the rough draft of your scholarship as you work out ideas and begin engaging in discussions with other profiles who have similar interests. These interactions go both ways. Not only will you need to post regularly, but you will need to engage other accounts. You get out of it what you put into it.

Table 8.1 Social media platforms

Name	Description	URL
Academia.edu	A self-described for profit open repository where scholars can share research with over 40 million pdfs.	Academia.edu: Share research
Figshare	An open access repository that adheres to the principles of open date where researchers can share research and other content.	https://figshare.com/
Mastodon	Mastodon is free and open-source software for running self-hosted social networking services. It has microblogging features similar to Twitter, which are offered by a large number of independently run nodes, known as instances, each with its own code of conduct, terms of service, privacy policy, privacy options, and content moderation policies. Instead of being a single, centralized place where everyone Tweets, replies, Mastodon is a decentralized network of individual servers. Each server is organized around a specific topic, company, or interest, and a server's members can interact with members of other servers.	https://mastodon.social/explore
Google Scholar	A search engine where researchers can find publications and track their own output with an account.	https://scholar.google.com/
Pinterest	An online vision board where you can share ideas and build concepts through sharing content.	https://www.pinterest.com/
Reddit	A large forum website where people with shared interests share information and have discussions.	https://www.reddit.com/
TikTok	A platform where users share short form videos.	https://www.tiktok.com/en/
YouTube	A video hosting website.	https://www.youtube.com/

General Guidelines and Best Practices

Scouting Content

The first step to curating your profile's information and the content you share is to do some preliminary research on similar accounts and areas of research. This can be helpful in two ways, One, you discover how your scholarship is being discussed and in turn you can find social media accounts to follow or include. This is where social media works as a two-way information exchange.

Well maintained and curated profiles will be the easiest to find and build relationships. If done well enough, other interested researchers will reach you.

Scouting tips:

- Explore hashtags on topics you are interested in.
- Look up regional and national associations related to your field.
- Look up libraries, schools, or institutions in your field.
- Look up other researchers who have given webinars or presentations.

Contribute Regularly

Regardless of the social media account, an active user will receive more engagement. However, the regularity in which you post depends on the platform. For some it may be beneficial to prepare a schedule, especially if you are writing your own content. A consistently posting profile will be perceived as more legitimate. In addition, you will have more sway over the content in your feed where you will see and interact with relevant accounts and people.

Save Your Hashtags#

On your scouting searches you will come across hashtags that may be interesting and link to relevant posts, and information. It is recommended you save some of these hashtags in a file. That way you can have them for reference later if you need help or want a quick and easy way to copy and paste hashtags that you use frequently.

Spelling Is Important

Luckily most social media platforms have a spell check feature. However, that sometimes comes in conflict with scholarly work since you may be working with concepts that are not recognized by the spell check software.

Emoji's

Use emojis sparingly. They can add some color and character but too much will overwhelm the post and clutter the message you are trying to convey [17].

Remain Courteous and Respectful

If you encounter a negative personality or become the target of mean malicious comments, you have the option to walk alway and not engage. You can then work to remove the offending profile or comments. You are completely in your right to block or delete interactions with negative people who do not seek any constructive criticism.

Celebrate Colleagues Accomplishments

Giving recognition to colleagues both on social media and in your workplace is one of the best uses of the platforms. Celebrate a poster presentation, a paper publication, or a successful project. Through encouragement we not only do a nice thing, but we also build a more positive environment that promotes scholarship.

Regulate Your Time on Social Media Platforms

The addictive properties of social media are well researched, and they can have a negative impact on your mental health and personality. It is important to put aside a block of time for interactions. This not only prevents information overload but can also help you manage what you can post.

Some platforms require more time than others, but a good rule of thumb is no more than 1 hour a day. If you find yourself exceeding this limit to your own determinant, an effective intervention is to place the device in another room, or out of sight. If that is not possible, completely logging out of the social account and not saving the password is an alternative. The concept behind the intervention is to put a barrier, physical or digital, between yourself and the account [27].

Bots

Watch out for Bots or "software robots." They are software systems designed to mimic human profiles. They exist in all social media platforms. Their goal is to manipulate the design of platforms to engage in users and build strong followings for multiple reasons including monetary gain, misinformation, or potential hacking [28]. They can mostly be avoided if you carefully curate your content and connections.

One Social Media Account Is Enough

As an individual, utilizing a single social media platform is enough. If you are looking to pick only one account for your scholarly profile, then select a platform with maximum visibility. In an academic setting LinkedIn is the priority platform. You have the most opportunity to make an impact and it will be the most likely place in which someone in your field of study will find you.

Conclusion

This information will help you get started in building your online digital presence through social media platforms. There are a variety of options to choose from and each one has their benefits, and one may suit your personality better than another. Don't get bogged down in trying to have accounts on all platforms, as it was mentioned previously one account is good enough. Most importantly, use these new connections to create a positive environment and support each other.

References

1. Bacev-Giles C, Haji R. Online first impressions: person perception in social media profiles. Comput Hum Behav. 2017;75:50–7. https://doi.org/10.1016/j.chb.2017.04.056.
2. Pew Research Center. Social Media fact sheet. 7 Apr 2021. https://www.pewresearch.org/internet/fact-sheet/social-media/. Accessed 20 Apr 2023.
3. Salik JR. From cynic to advocate: the use of Twitter in cardiology. J Am Coll Cardiol. 2020;76(5):623–7. https://doi.org/10.1016/j.jacc.2020.06.050.

4. Nicholas D, Boukacem-Zeghmouri C, Rodríguez-Bravo B, Xu J, Watkinson A, Abrizah A, Herman E, Świgoń M. Where and how early career researchers find scholarly information. Learn Publ. 2017;30(1):19–29. https://doi.org/10.1002/leap.1087.
5. Prabhu V, Lovett JT, Munawar K. Role of social and non-social online media: how to properly leverage your internet presence for professional development and research. Abdom Radiol (NY). 2021;46(12):5513–20. https://doi.org/10.1007/s00261-021-03154-0.
6. Abbot L. 10 Tips for taking a professional LinkedIn profile photo. LinkedIn. 2022. https://www.linkedin.com/business/talent/blog/product-tips/tips-for-taking-professional-linkedin-profile-pictures. Accessed 20 Apr 2023.
7. Clark S. Degrees of LinkedIn Connection. LinkedIn. 2016. https://www.linkedin.com/pulse/degrees-linkedin-connection-sid-clark/. Accessed 20 Apr 2023.
8. LinkedIn Groups Membership: overview. 2022. https://www.linkedin.com/help/linkedin/answer/a540824/groups-getting-started?lang=en. Accessed 20 Apr 2023.
9. Marr B. Big data in practice: how 45 successful companies used big data analytics to deliver extraordinary results. Oxford: John Wiley & Sons; 2016.
10. Dehan J. 20 steps to a better LinkedIn profile in 2023. LinkedIn Best Practices. 2023. https://www.linkedin.com/business/sales/blog/profile-best-practices/17-steps-to-a-better-linkedin-profile-in-2017. Accessed 20 Apr 2023.
11. Lowes P. The ultimate LinkedIn post type guide. 2020. https://www.linkedin.com/pulse/ultimate-linkedin-post-type-guide-peter-lowes/. Accessed 20 Apr 2023.
12. O'Brien K. ResearchGate. J Med Library Assoc. 2019;107(2):284–5. https://doi.org/10.5195/jmla.2019.643.
13. Kwon D. ResearchGate dealt a blow in copyright lawsuit. Nature. 2022;603:375–6. https://doi.org/10.1038/d41586-022-00513-9.
14. ResearchGate. 2023. https://www.researchgate.net/. Accessed 20 Apr 2023.
15. Doyle A. Office of Career Services. Mignone Center for Career Success. Harvard University Faculty of Arts and Science. How to give a great elevator pitch. 2022. https://careerservices.fas.harvard.edu/blog/2022/10/11/how-to-create-an-elevator-pitch-with-examples. Accessed 23 Apr 2023.
16. Keutelian M. The best times to post on social media in 2022. Sprout Social. 29 Mar 2023. https://sproutsocial.com/insights/best-times-to-post-on-social-media/. Accessed 19 Apr 2023.
17. Rzewnicki D. Tips and tricks on how to use Twitter. BMJ. 2021;375:n2225. https://doi.org/10.1136/bmj.n2225.
18. How to protect and unprotect your tweets | twitter help. Twitter. 2023. https://help.twitter.com/en/safety-and-security/how-to-make-twitter-private-and-public. Accessed 20 Apr 2023.
19. Global Instagram User Age & Gender Distribution 2023. Statista. 14 Feb 2023. https://www.statista.com/statistics/248769/age-distribution-of-worldwide-instagram-users/. Accessed 20 Apr 2023.
20. Doney J, Wikle O, Martinez J. Likes, comments, views: a content analysis of academic library Instagram posts. Inf Technol Libr. 2020;39(3) https://doi.org/10.6017/ital.v39i3.12211.
21. Cooper P. The best time to post on Instagram in 2023 [complete guide]. Social Media Marketing & Management Dashboard. 5 Jan 2023. https://blog.hootsuite.com/best-time-to-post-on-instagram/. Accessed 20 Apr 2023.
22. Moreau E. 12 Instagram tips for Beginners. Lifewire. 25 June 2021. https://www.lifewire.com/instagram-tips-for-beginners-3485872. Accessed 20 Apr 2023.
23. Share of Facebook users in the United States as of March 2023, by age group. Statista. 11 Apr 2023. https://www.statista.com/statistics/187549/facebook-distribution-of-users-age-group-usa/. Accessed 20 Apr 2023.
24. Meisenzahl M. The 16 biggest scandals Mark Zuckerberg faced over the last decade as he became one of the world's most powerful people. Business Insider. 3 Nov 2021. https://www.businessinsider.com/mark-zuckerberg-scandals-last-decade-while-running-facebook-2019-12. Accessed 20 Apr 2023.

25. Hall M. Facebook. Encyclopedia Britannica. 29 Mar 2023. https://www.britannica.com/topic/Facebook.
26. Your profile: Facebook help center. Facebook. 2023. https://www.facebook.com/help/396528481579093/?helpref=hc_fnav. Accessed 20 Apr 2023.
27. Biedermann D, Schneider J, Drachsler H. Digital self-control interventions for distracting media multitasking: a systematic review. J Comput Assist Learn. 2021;37(5):1217–31. https://doi.org/10.1111/jcal.12581.
28. Orabi M, Mouheb D, Al Aghbari Z, Kamel I. Detection of bots in social media: a systematic review. Inf Process Manag. 2020;57(4):102250. https://doi.org/10.1016/j.ipm.2020.102250.

Chapter 9
Risks, Privacy, and Harassment

Margaret Rush Dreker

Introduction

Social media and online platforms are useful tools for academics and researchers. These outlets are used for creation, dissemination, collaboration, communication, and other academic pursuits. For students, researchers, scientists, or academics these platforms can highlight research interests, measure research impact, and act as a forum to share and learn new ideas. Social media platforms in the twenty-first century can be compared to the twentieth century conference or professional meeting. It is a space to meet, network, and to share academic pursuits.

Research collaborations have expanded and grown by the sharing of information on digital academic platforms such as ORCID, Scopus, Web of Science, and Research Gate [1]. Using digital tools, researchers can quickly identify individuals or groups working in the same field which can lead to collaborative research projects.

During the COVID-19 pandemic the growth of misinformation on social network platforms [2] spread exponentially. It is virtually impossible to turn the tide on misinformation, but scientists, researchers and academics use their digital presence to dispel the myths and misinformation.

One problem with this new role of having a platform to share ideas quickly is there is no way to verify an individual's credentials on social media; no official check mark is offered such as on Twitter or X. [3]. Fake profiles can easily be established, and misinformation spread. Having a reputable "digital identity" is important during a time of mass information communication. It takes 20 years to build a reputation and few minutes of a cyber incident to ruin it.

M. R. Dreker (✉)
Hackensack Meridian School of Medicine, Nutley, NJ, USA
e-mail: Margaret.dreker@hmhn.org

© The Author(s), under exclusive license to Springer Nature Switzerland AG 2023
M. R. Dreker, K. J. Downey (eds.), *Building Your Academic Research Digital Identity*, https://doi.org/10.1007/978-3-031-50317-7_9

Social media platforms have changed the way we communicate. While these platforms present true opportunities for academics and researchers, they also come with risks. As with all social media there are privacy concerns, harassment, identity theft and plagiarism. All of these revolve around the main concern of "reputation." Any misuse of social media can cause irreputable harm to the individual and destroy a career for a researcher. Research can be misinterpreted on social media ruining a lifelong career. This also makes a teacher, a professor, or a researcher a candidate for harassment, targeted violence, and stalking.

First Steps Before Establishing a Digital Profile

Avoiding social media altogether is not possible or realistic in the world of academics or research. Establishing a digital profile is the first step in finding a balance between the benefits and risks of online activity and how to deal with problems if they arise.

The following list are things that should always be assumed before setting up a digital presence on any social media platform:

- No one is anonymous on any social media platform.
- Nothing is private.
- Once something is posted on a social media site it spreads quickly.
- Everyone can see what you post.
- An embarrassing comment, post, or image will come back to haunt you.
- The more you participate in social media platforms, the higher your risk is for harassment, identity theft and other behaviors.

Profile Pictures

Most social media platforms available to academics allow for a profile picture or head shot to be uploaded. When others visit your site, they expect to see a photo associated with the user profile. A profile picture can be vital in establishing your personal brand or the university brand you represent.

There are a few options when choosing a photo. The university or organization may have workplace social media policies that define what type of photo may be uploaded. A professional headshot is the best option to be uploaded to any platform (Fig. 9.1).

Each digital platform has guidelines for an uploaded picture or headshot.

Using the same photo across all platforms will make you more recognizable and raise your visibility. Do not change your profile picture often since people will recognize your profile image while scrolling through your posts.

Social Media Platform	Head Shot Requirements
LinkedIn	Horizontal images to company page or personal profile: 1,104 x 736 pixels
Twitter	Single horizontal image: 1,200 x 675 pixels
Facebook	1,200 x 630 pixels for horizontal images.

Fig. 9.1 Head shot and image size requirements [4]

The profile picture is your first chance to communicate that you are friendly, likable, and trustworthy. All attributes that are crucial to getting others to engage with you. It is your first step to building your personal brand on many platforms.

Many social media platforms do not allow profile pictures to be hidden from public view in the same way that you can restrict other images you publish.

Cover and profile images on Twitter or X are always publicly visible. Facebook also states that your profile picture and cover photo are always public, specifically so that people can recognize you (and this extends to details such as your gender, age range, and networks). LinkedIn provides the option of changing the profile picture's public visibility, but the default option is that the image can be seen by anyone. The required photo may be a reason while some researchers chose not to use this platform.

Risks of Using a Profile Picture

There are security risks associated with using a profile picture on any platform, so many people chose to use an alias profile picture. This can cause problems since facial recognition tools are publicly available. Facial recognition creates another complication to posting profile pictures.

If using a simple Chrome browser, you can right click on any profile picture, and it will provide links to all matching and similar images in Google. The default Twitter or X profile image is associated with "bots" and if someone comes across your profile, they may be less likely to interact with you for fear or follow you thinking you may be a bot [5].

Some platforms are now using facial recognition systems to biometrically profile and identify millions of faces. The face in the profile picture must be recognized as the same people viewing it and by the platforms algorithms [4].

Profile pictures are often indexed by search engines, where they can be accessed and copied by anyone, regardless of whether they are members of that platform. From a stalker looking for details about a person's whereabouts, to a company looking for compromising information on an employee or rival, it's easy to imagine how these kinds of tools can end up being abused.

More professional images are likely to show you in a way in which you can be easily identified. Universities and organizations may use these on "About Us" or "Meet the Team" or the "Library Staff" pages. Because of this, you may not always have permissions over where and how your profile images are used, but the more an image is used online the greater the risk of it being stolen and used without your consent.

Others may use your images on fake profiles so people may attribute anything found on that false profile to you. This could be in the forms of scams, fraudulent offers, pornographic material, requests for money, plagiarism, or online trolls. Having a profile picture on this fake account now places these undesirable actions under the umbrella of your face and image.

Some images will naturally be less susceptible to theft than others, such as those that don't show the individual clearly. This could be because the subject is at a distance or occupies a small portion of the image for some other reason, or perhaps because they are wearing a pair of sunglasses or a hat that obscures certain facial details.

The best advice is to keep just one professional profile picture for all social media accounts which will limit the availability of pictures to steal and keep it connected to just your profile.

Plagiarism

Plagiarism is pervasive in the academic sector. Plagiarism has been committed by students and by academics; the topic of plagiarism has been frequently raised at meetings, at educational institutions and research organizations all over the world (Fig. 9.2).

Fig. 9.2: Best practice to secure your digital profile [6]

- Do not accept friend/follow requests from anyone you do not know.
- Avoid third party applications.
- Be cautious with the images you post. Utilize the same professional headshot for all platforms.
- Configure your security options on your accounts to minimize who can see your information.
- Never check "Remember Me" or "Keep Me Logged In" option from a public or shared computer.
- Do not use the same passwords for all your accounts.
- Do not use your social media accounts to log into other sites.
- Utilize privacy settings to manage your profile.

Fig. 9.3 Best practices if you discover you are a victim of plagiarism: [8]

- Get a screen capture, URL, and all other available information about the offending content right away.
- File a DMCA complaint (Digital Millennium Copyright Act). This act criminalizes copyright infringement.
- Confront your Plagiarist in person.
- Get the word out.
- Use the Rel=Author tag in the html of your online content.

Plagiarism occurs when one writer attempts to pass off another writer's work as their own [7]. But that's not all plagiarism is. Plagiarism also occurs when a writer references another's work in their own writing and doesn't properly credit the author whose work they referenced. It's even possible for a writer to plagiarize their own work without citations. Writing is work, and it can be very challenging work at times. Claiming somebody else's work as your own strips them of the recognition they deserve for the effort they put into creating it and gives yourself undue credit.

Plagiarism in academia is a well-known problem; and both students and professors can be guilty of stealing another person's work. Professors and research supervisors stealing unsuspecting doctoral student intellectual property has happened many times. There have even been stories of the clever person who translates work from foreign languages, and no one, including the original author is aware (Fig. 9.3).

So, don't be surprised to find your research published under your colleague's or someone else's name. There are numerous examples and court cases of plagiarism and mismanagement of research data resulting in leaked research by careless supervisors and untrusting researchers.

Having all your personal information online and available makes plagiarism easier to accomplish.

Predatory authors develop when an undeserving scientists impose themselves as coauthors on other people's papers. All these predatory activities serve the purpose of padding one's Curriculum Vitae or CV. The more digital information about a researcher that is available and the wider dissemination of their work over social media platforms, the more likely to have their work stolen. Peer review digitization has also allowed exposure of instances of stealing ideas and materials which are intended for confidential and privileged evaluation by reviewers [7].

"In 2015, academic journal publisher Elsevier, retracted nine articles because the cases involved authors posing as their own peer reviewers, a new and emerging trend of identity fraud which, by far, is the most serious in recent years," Philippe Terheggen, Elsevier's Managing Director of STM Journals, told Science & Technology Daily in an interview [9].

In this case, the authors suggested peer reviewers. It turns out those suggested peer reviewers were the authors themselves. The fraud was exposed by checking academic profiles and comparing email addresses from the Scopus author profile feature. Stricter publication standards have since been put in place.

Cyber Bullying

Occupation is a significant factor in the case of harassment in the adult population. Attention should be given to especially vulnerable professional groups such as politicians, academics, and other knowledge workers who are most exposed to the public due to their occupation [10]. The recent rise of anti-intellectualism paved the way for academics to become hate speech targets in a manner similar to how political beliefs or social status can increase an individual's risk for online victimization [10]. Having access through digital identity platforms makes that harassment a lot simpler and that much more anonymous.

A Pew Research Center survey of U.S. adults in September 2021 finds that 41% of Americans have personally experienced some form of online harassment in at least one of the six key ways that were measured. And while the overall prevalence of this type of abuse is the same as it was in 2017, there is evidence that online harassment has intensified since then.

Growing shares of Americans report experiencing more severe forms of harassment, which encompasses physical threats, stalking, sexual harassment, and sustained harassment. Some 15% experienced such problems in 2014 and a slightly larger share (18%) said the same in 2017. Today that group has risen to 25%. Additionally, those who have been the target of online abuse are more likely today, than in 2017, to report that their most recent experience involved more varied types and more severe forms of online abuse [11].

Cyber bullying is bullying that takes place over digital devices such as cell phones, computers, and tablets. Cyberbullying can occur through SMS, text and apps, or in online social media, forums, or gaming where people can view, participate in, or share content. Cyberbullying includes sending, posting, or sharing negative, harmful, false, or mean content about someone else. It can include sharing personal or private information about someone else causing embarrassment or humiliation. Some cyberbullying crosses the line into unlawful or criminal behavior [12].

With the prevalence of social media and digital forums, comments, photos, posts, and content shared by individuals can often be viewed by strangers as well as colleagues. The content an individual shares online—both their personal content as well as any negative, mean, or hurtful content—creates a permanent public record of their views, activities, and behavior. This public record can be thought of as an online reputation, which may be accessible to schools, employers, colleges, clubs, and others who may be researching an individual now or in the future.

Indeed, 20% of Americans overall—representing half of those who have been harassed online—say they have experienced online harassment because of their political views. This is a notable increase from 3 years ago, when 14% of all Americans said they had been targeted for this reason. Beyond politics, more also cite their gender or their racial and ethnic background as reasons why they believe they were harassed online [11].

Cyberbullying can harm the online reputations of everyone involved—not just the person being bullied, but those doing the bullying or participating in it.

Damaging a reputation has long term repercussions in hiring, publishing, grants and promotion and tenure. Course enrollment may impact evaluations and pay. Low enrolled classes might be canceled leaving an instructor out of a position or with a pay cut. Additionally, on other social media sites such as "Rate My Professor" the negative comments can be used as an unofficial resource that influences official decisions about hiring, pay, and tenure. Many professors are left powerless if a disgruntled student use this social platform to smear their reputation. Defamatory comments on professor-rating sites remain in place for all future students to see. There have been cases of colleagues also using this rating platform to anonymously hurt a colleagues' reputation.

Online Harassment

Researchers using social media platforms and academic platforms maybe asked to speak publicly on topics, many of which are not popular. Those conducting research into sensitive topics may face online harassment. This was on full display during the COVID-19 pandemic [13]. Two surveys of scientists' experiences of harassment during the pandemic, from personal insults to death threats, suggest a dispiriting, if unsurprising, trend: researchers with greater news-media prominence are more likely to be harassed.

In March 2022, Science's news team reported that 38% of researchers who have published multiple papers on COVID-19 said they had experienced at least one type of harassment related to their COVID-19 work [14]. In a 2021 Nature news survey of over 300 scientists, 81% of respondents said that they had experienced personal attacks or trolling—even if only rarely—after talking to the media about COVID-19. And 70% reported at least one kind of negative impact after speaking to the media or posting on social media, ranging from receiving physical threats to experiencing emotional distress [15].

Researchers studying climate change, gender studies, politics, and other topics have been targets of online harassment. Varied scientists, spokespersons, and researchers reported continued levels of harassment through social media platforms. In the 2021 Nature survey, more than two-thirds of researchers reported negative experiences as a result of their media appearances or their social media comments, and 22% had received threats of physical or sexual violence. Some scientists said that their employer had received complaints about them, or that their home address had been revealed online. Six scientists said they were physically attacked [15].

This online harassment can lead to more severe forms of harassment and may even pose physical danger to the researcher. False, misrepresented, or private information propagated by harassers may negatively impact the researcher's reputation and/or career. If the researcher goes to their institution seeking help, their concerns may be ignored, misunderstood, or not taken seriously. Ultimately, fear of harassment may have a negative effect on the type of research that is conducted and the capabilities of individual researchers [6].

One way that individuals may harass a researcher is by bombarding their institution with messages, complaints, and threats—even if those complaints are empty and without merit—in a coordinated attempt to discredit them or get them fired. Individuals may recruit additional people or create fake accounts to make online harassment look like legitimate public outcry, or to seem like a significant threat to an institution's reputation. Online harassment campaigns can vary widely in terms of scale and duration. They are meant to damage the standing of the researcher within their institution; impede their research; damage their public character; or challenge the validity of their work.

Beyond direct harassment of the researcher, examples of online harassment relevant to institutions or universities include complaints and threats about the researcher to the institution's social media accounts; emails or phone calls to institutional review boards, department chairs, or deans; and harassment of the researcher's colleagues or affiliates.

Doxing, is a form of online harassment used to exact revenge and to threaten and destroy the privacy of individuals by making their personal information public, including addresses, social security, credit card and phone numbers, links to social media accounts, and other private data. Doxing can be a coordinated social media campaign and threatening emails or phone calls to scientists and their employers. While doxing itself is not illegal, it may fall under stalking and harassment laws, depending on where you live and the degree of harassment.

Online Hate: Race and Gender

Online hate (i.e., cyberhate, online hate speech) is an expression of hatred or prejudice toward a group of people based on specific group characteristics, for example their ethnicity, religion, or sexual orientation [10]. Women and minorities have been the groups mostly subject to online harassment. Online harassment is an issue that disproportionately affects women, as they "experience a wider variety of online abuse, including more serious violations" than men [16]. A 2018 Amnesty International (AI) study, across eight countries, found that 23% of women experienced online abuse or harassment. Another found that the number of women who reported being sexually harassed online had doubled since their last survey in 2017 [17].

There are several demographic differences regarding who has been harassed online for their gender or their race or ethnicity. Among adults who have been harassed online, roughly half of women (47%) say they think they have encountered harassment online because of their gender, whereas 18% of men who have been harassed online say the same. Similarly, about half or more Black (54%) or Hispanic online harassment targets (47%) say they were harassed due to their race or ethnicity, compared with 17% of white targets [11].

In a 2012 study of 524 professors, from 100 colleges and universities across the USA were surveyed, it was found that women, People of Color, LGBTQ+ faculty, younger faculty, and newer faculty reported more incivility from students than their white male counterparts [18]. Research has shown that male students were more likely to engage in vengeful dissent and behaviors [19].

Problematic online behaviors can include trolling, insults, sexual harassment, rape and death threats, are frequently compounded with racism, homophobia, ableism, and all other forms of hate [17]. This online abuse can influence women's digital presence and constrain a women's willingness to speak on their individual research or how they speak publicly about other academic topics.

Colleague on Colleague Online Harassment

Power imbalances are prevalent in the hierarchical of all universities and research labs. Administrator to faculty member, senior to junior faculty, tenured to untenured, faculty to staff, supervisor to graduate student, instructor to student, not to mention imbalances based on gender, age, ethnicity, race, social status, and sexual orientation, which can permeate all of those relationships [20]. These relationships can lead to the exercise of power and control over another in a relationship and lead to abuses such as cyber bullying.

Cassidy found that lesbian, gay, bisexual, and queer (LGBTQ+) faculty and staff are more likely to experience bullying in the university workplace from superiors, colleagues, and subordinates, highlighting the interplay of gender, race, ethnicity, and sexuality (intersectionality) when it comes to bullying [20]. Lampman [18] found that women, minorities, younger faculty, those with less experience and credentials are more likely to be targets of bullying and online harassment.

Faculty members feel if they did complain that they risked being seen as the problem could impact their reputation as well as their ability to advance in the university or research organization.

How to Handle Harassment

Pulling back from online engagement can be especially damaging for researchers, whose online presence is often important for their careers. Informing the necessary people of the harassment is important to do immediately. Keep evidence of cyberbullying. Record the dates, times, and descriptions of instances when cyberbullying has occurred. Save and print screenshots, emails, and text messages. Use this evidence to report cyberbullying to web and cell phone service providers. Your institution will be able to offer security and safety if complaints are filed about your research through social media.

Trolling

Trolling is when a person posts or writes degrading, hateful, mean, and inflammatory statements that are intentionally defamatory to "bait" someone into a response. Trolling is primarily done in spaces deliberately set up for others to see and even engage in trolling behavior. The comments and remarks of the trolling cyber bullies are often directed at the faculty member's superior by providing content deliberately trying to cause some type of punishment or distress to the faculty.

As a researcher, you should limit your response to individuals during this time. It is a natural human instinct to defend oneself when being attacked. By engaging with their insults or threats, you are giving them exactly what they want. Therefore, whenever possible, it is best to stay silent and not risk escalating a situation. Universities or organizations that encourage social media platform communication will have to support the researchers when harassment occurs. If your research is grant funded, you should inform the funding organization of the social media harassment.

Cyberbullying often violates the terms of service established by social media sites and internet service providers. Review their terms and conditions or rights and responsibilities sections. These describe content that is or is not appropriate. Report cyberbullying to the social media site so they can take action against users abusing the terms of service. Twitter or X has an Abusive Behavior Policy, which states:

> You may not engage in the targeted harassment of someone or incite other people to do so. We consider abusive behavior an attempt to harass, intimidate, or silence someone else's voice [21].

Penalties for violation of the platforms policies included deleting the inflammatory Tweet or being blocked from the platform.

The ORCID Code of Conduct [22] states;

> Behavior that reflects our values is required across all internal and external interactions and communications. We recognize that professional behavior that embodies our values precludes and prohibits abuses of power. We commit to taking disciplinary action, including at our discretion termination of employment, contract, or affiliation in response to any verified acts of harassment, bullying, intimidation, discrimination, or other serious breach of this Code of Conduct, made by any member of staff against anyone and all members of the ORCID community, and with other staff members. We also expect our vendors, contractors, consultants, members, and partners to abide by all of these commitments in their interactions with ORCID.

If all else fails and the harassment gets to be too much, don't hesitate to block the users account, and file a report through the proper channels. Every social media platform has a procedure for reporting users who violate the company's code of conduct. It may take a few days for the company to do its due diligence. However, if the situation is quickly escalating, contact support—they may offer a helpful solution in many cases.

When cyber bullying involves threats of violence, sexually explicit photos, video, or pictures of someone in a place where he or she would expect privacy and stalking or hate crimes, the police should be called. If anyone online threatens your property or safety, you want to report it to the police in addition to the social media platform. Although they may not be able to act on the report, this creates a paper trail, so you have formal documentation in the event that the social media harassment escalates.

File a report with the police where your university and home are located and include all documentation of harassment or cyberstalking. If you have evidence of the perpetrator's identity, file a restraining order because you don't know when that person might take the harassment offline.

Before establishing any digital profile or social media accounts you should:

- Be aware of the internal mechanisms of the platform that address online harassment. How do you report harassment, can you block an individual, is the platform content moderated?
- Working with a friend, send harassing materials to your profiles and social media accounts to see if you receive any notifications of the harassing behavior.
- Discuss issues of academic freedom with your university or organization's office of research so you understand the steps in reporting harassment, and you understand the support that will be offered by the university or organization.
- Ensure all your profile and social media accounts are protected by strong passwords.
- Review all accounts and see who is "following" you or is a "friend" and delete unknow accounts.
- Set up two-factor authentication on any email accounts and social media accounts.
- Remove your personal address, phone numbers from any public CV's or resumes.
- Consider setting up an "alias email" which points to your direct email during this harassment.
- Run a Google search and see where your personal information, address, phone number, may be listed.

Researchers and academics may face harassment and abuse when their views and research is posted on digital platforms. Dr. Anthony Fauci, who became the face of the 2019 COVID pandemic with his daily television updates, even spoke out against "low-life" trolls harassing his wife and children, figuring out where they live and their phone numbers. In a December 2022, BBC podcast, Dr. Fauci stated he tries his best not to be distracted by online hate that "takes away from your ability to do your job" [23].

Knowledge of the platforms used to establish your digital identity, familiarity with the privacy settings, establishment of secure passwords, and knowledge of your organizations social media guidelines will be the first steps in providing a secure online space for researchers.

Conclusion

Research has shown that student-to-faculty cyberbullying is a problem in higher education, causing even larger burdens on faculty. One of the major problems is that universities and other academic institutions have focused on keeping their students safe, while assuming faculty and researchers are exempt from or immune to cyber bullying.

Many institutions have little or no support to assist faculty facing any form of online cyber harassment from students. Just like other forms of harassment, online harassment victims can feel unsupported by their superiors or the university. It seems many universities are not providing enough support, avenues of reporting, or counseling for faculty victims of cyberbullying. Checking whether an institution has a grievance policy or faculty senate that can offer support to those who have been bullied online can be helpful.

If you are being harassed online, reaching out to your co-workers, peers and professional colleagues can be helpful since they can offer support. They may have also faced a similar experience and may offer support or suggestions. Unions can also offer advice in dealing with this situation. Another step may be to consult with the university's ombudsman or an equivalent office. These offices exist at most large research institutions, in the USA and around the world, to offer an informal, impartial, and confidential conflict-management service that operates independently of the university.

It is okay to feel frustrated, isolated, or anxious about the harassment you have been facing. If you are feeling stressed, talk to a friend or a professional to help work through your feelings. Harassment is a major trauma.

Online harassment directed at researchers can hinder the perceived value of clinical research, which in turn halts new development by restricting scientists' access to funds and other resources. This online harassment can influence the quality of public discussion and it can lead to researchers' imposing limitations and restrictions on their digital platforms as a way of avoiding abuse. Online harassment may also negatively influence scholars' relationships with social media and cut out that important line of communication with other scholars.

For researchers and faculty to continue to effectively grow and develop, institutions must be supportive and provide the safest workplace possible.

Resources for Combatting Online Harassment

Crash Override: http://www.crashoverridenetwork.com/
Crash Override is a crisis helpline, advocacy group, and resource center for people experiencing online abuse. They are a network of experts and survivors who work directly with individuals, tech companies, media, security experts, and law enforcement to educate and provide direct assistance.

HeartMob: https://iheartmob.org/
A private platform that provides community support for people experiencing online harassment.

Internet Matters.Org: https://www.internetmatters.org/issues/cyberbullying/resources/
Resources to help combat Cyberbullying. Internet Matters is a non-profit organization with the goal of keeping kids safe online. These tips can be used to also help adults protect themselves against cyberbullying.

National Network to End Domestic Violence Technology Safety Resources: https://nnedv.org/content/technology-safety/
A collection of resources to help individuals and agencies respond effectively to the many ways in which technology impacts victims of domestic and dating violence, sexual violence, and stalking.

Speak Up and Stay Safe: A Guide to Protecting Yourself from Online Harassment: https://feministfrequency.com/2015/12/08/speak-up-stay-safer-a-guide-to-protecting-yourself-from-online-harassment/
A fantastic, detailed guide on how to protect yourself online from the creators of Feminist Frequency and Women, Action and the Media.

Violet Blue, The Smart Girl's Guide to Privacy (No Starch Press, 2015) 978-1593276485.
A great short book that covers many of the issues in this document in more depth.

Without My Consent: https://withoutmyconsent.org/
Without My Consent is a non-profit organization seeking to combat online invasions of privacy. Their resources are intended to empower individuals to stand up for their privacy rights and inspire meaningful debate about accountability, free speech, and the internet.

Zen and the Art of Making Tech Work for You: https://tacticaltech.org/news/zen-resource/
A manual for managing online presence and creating safe spaces online, by the Tactical Technology Collective.

References

1. Hoang DT, Nguyen NT, Tran VC, Hwang D. Research collaboration model in academic social networks. Enterp Inf Syst. 2019;13(7–8):1023–45. https://doi.org/10.1080/17517575.2018.1556812.
2. Skafle I, Nordahl-Hansen A, Quintana DS, Wynn R, Gabarron E. Misinformation about COVID-19 vaccines on social media: rapid review. J Med Internet Res. 2022;24(8):e37367. https://doi.org/10.2196/37367.
3. Twitter: What does the blue checkmark mean? 2022. https://help.twitter.com/en/managing-your-account/about-twitter-verified-accounts. Accessed 12 Dec 2022.

4. Ntrepid: profile pictures on social media. 2022. https://ntrepidcorp.com/managed-attribution/social-media-profile-pics-operational-risks/. Accessed 3 Feb 2023.
5. Allen K, Jimerson S, Quintana D, McKinley L. An academic's guide to social media learn, engage, and belong. New York: Routledge; 2023.
6. Marwick A, Blackwell L, Lo K. Best practices for conducting risky research. New York: Data & Society Research institute; 2016.
7. Zimba O, Gasparyan A. Plagiarism detection and prevention: a primer for researchers. Reumatologia. 2021;59(3):132–7. https://doi.org/10.5114/reum.2021.105974.
8. Kendall J. Fighting plagiarism 101. 2012. https://www.socialmediatoday.com/content/fighting-plagiarism-101. Accessed Mar 2023.
9. Chan J. China reins in on identity fraud over concerns of author, reviewer authenticity. 2015. https://www.elsevier.com/connect/china-reigns-in-on-identity-fraud-over-concerns-of-author-reviewer-authenticity. Accessed 1 Mar 2023.
10. Celuch M, Savela N, Oksa R, Latikka R, Oksanen A. Individual factors predicting reactions to online harassment among finnish professionals. Comput Hum Behav. 2022;127:107022. https://doi.org/10.1016/j.chb.2021.107022.
11. Vogels E. The state of online-harassment 2021. Pew Charitable Trust Foundation. 2021.
12. Stop Bullying. 2023. www.stopbullying.gov. Accessed 3 Feb 2023.
13. O'Grady C. In the line of fire. Science. 2022;375(6587):1338.
14. Van Noorden R. Higher-profile COVID experts more likely to get online abuse. Nature. 2022; https://doi.org/10.1038/d41586-022-00936-4.
15. Nogrady B. 'I hope you die': how the COVID pandemic unleashed attacks on scientists. Nature. 2021;598(7880):250–3. https://doi.org/10.1038/d41586-021-02741-x.
16. Gelms B. Social media research and the methodological problem of harassment: foregrounding researcher safety. Comput Compos. 2021;59:102626. https://doi.org/10.1016/j.compcom.2021.102626.
17. Amensty International. Toxic Twitter: triggers of violence and abuse against women on Twitter. 2018.
18. Lampman C. Women faculty at risk: U.S. professors report on their experiences with student incivility, bullying, aggression, and sexual attention. NASPA J Women High Educ. 2012;5(5):184–208. https://doi.org/10.1515/njawhe-2012-1108.
19. Goodboy AK, Myers SA. Instructional dissent as an expression of students' verbal aggressiveness and argumentativeness traits. Commun Educ. 2012;61(4):448–58. https://doi.org/10.1080/03634523.2012.699635.
20. Cassidy W, Faucher C, Jackson M. Adversity in university: cyberbullying and its impacts on students, faculty and administrators. Int J Environ Res Public Health. 2017;14(8):888. https://doi.org/10.3390/ijerph14080888.
21. Twitter: abusive behavior. 2023. https://help.twitter.com/en/rules-and-policies/abusive-behavior. Accessed Jan 2023.
22. ORCID Open Researcher and Contributor IDentifier: ORCID code of conduct. https://info.orcid.org/code-of-conduct/. Accessed 12 Dec 2022.
23. Spring M. PA. Dr Anthony Fauci Talks: Covid, China and Online Misinformation. BBC Americast. 2022.

Chapter 10
Mapping Out Your Digital Presence

Kyle James Downey and Margaret Rush Dreker

Flow of Misinformation and Digital Identities

Will the spread of misinformation be slowed by the growth of digital profiles and identifiers? Researchers and academics should only make statements on social media and other platforms that are based on evidence to support those claims. Knowledge sources should be transparent and clearly communicated whether verbally or in writing. Having a digital profile allows transparency so the author and their credentials are clearly identifiable to others on that platform.

Social Ethics

The social and ethical issues raised in relation to privacy, data mining, and subsequent use of information gathered from ASNSs and social platforms warrant attention. As a user, it is your responsibility to understand the privacy and data collection policies of each platform on which you have a digital profile. Digital platform users have all agreed to a set of terms and conditions for each platform, and within these terms and conditions there are often clauses on how one's data may be accessed by third parties, including researchers.

K. J. Downey (✉)
College of Nursing & School of Health and Medical Sciences Librarian, Seton Hall University, Nutley, NJ, USA
e-mail: kyle.downey@shu.edu

M. R. Dreker
Hackensack Meridian School of Medicine, Nutley, NJ, USA
e-mail: Margaret.dreker@hmhn.org

This emphasizes the importance of ownership and consent to protect your digital identity and professional reputation.

Privacy

As an academic joining a digital platform, it is important to protect your information and maintain how it is controlled or shared. To do that:

- Review the privacy settings of a platform. This allows you to control who can see your profile information, how much information is being shared and with whom.
- Is the data you wish to access on an open forum or platform—Is it located within a closed or private group or a closed discussion forum?
- Is the group or forum password protected?
- Does the group have a moderator or administrator that you could turn to for approval and advice?

Use your account privacy settings to control (as much as possible) how others' online activities can affect your visibility. Don't rely on the user default privacy settings of any platform. They get changed periodically. Carefully review privacy policies, and update your settings periodically, proactively, and strategically [1].

Infrastructure

Universities and other research institutions will have to invest in reliable and secure online digital platforms. This would help ensure that online learning sessions, and other online engagements are not disrupted by technical issues. Technical support should be made available to both academics and students to help identify and address any issues that arise. Schools and universities should provide technical support staff or contact information to help troubleshoot any technical issues that may arise using digital platforms. Organizations will also have to provide training and support to help develop digital literacy skills of students, faculty, and researchers. This could be in the form of webinars, tutorials, and courses that cover topics such as online communication etiquette, privacy, and faculty rights and responsibilities in an academic environment.

Promotion and Tenure

What effect will having a digital presence on social media or ASNS have on researchers and academics on the tenure track? Will digital scholarship play a role in academic advancement, promotion or tenure?

Tenure is a rank earned by scholars working at the university level who have completed a set probationary period at their institution, usually 5–7 years, and have been awarded this position by a review committee made up of their faculty dean, department chair, and a selection of their peers. This status is an important achievement; as after the attainment of a tenured faculty position at an institution, a scholar cannot be fired or let go without proven adequate cause.

To earn tenure, a faculty member must meet certain requirements as set out by their institution. These requirements are usually separated into three broad components: (1) Research, (2) Service, and (3) Teaching. Although these components are usually given equal weight in the tenure and promotion review process, each component may vary from one academic institution to another.

The research component of the tenure review process can include a wide range of activities, including scholars' reputation in their field, conference participation, and originality of research. Traditionally, scholarly output in the form of a peer-reviewed journal article has been at the core of committee deliberations, looking at publication metrics such as the journal's prestige (measured by its impact factor), and the number of citations, among others [2].

Despite the current lack of official support by the scholarly community, some academic institutions are beginning to see the importance of social media and networking sites and are beginning to advocate for its use. In early 2016, the Mayo Clinic Academic Appointments and Promotions Committee began including digital and social media scholarship among the criteria considered in review of proposals for academic advancement [3].

One of the reasons why so few institutions explicitly do not endorse digital/social media for promotion is because there is no consensus about what constitutes digital and social media scholarship appropriate for promotion, in terms of which formats merit inclusion, or how to assess quality, though efforts are underway to create benchmarks [2].

Publishers of scholarly journals are also increasingly adding social media and networking capabilities to their digital resources. Publishers are not only using online social media themselves but are developing ways to measure scholars' impact in the realm of online social media. Publishers have developed ways to measure the number of times an article are bookmarked, viewed, and the number of mentions of the article on online social media sites such as blogs.

As a response to the traditional impact-based system, a new set of tools has emerged. Altmetrics seeks to measure the impact of research output beyond the academic world. It is gaining acceptance, as an increasing number of academics contribute to scholarship via digital means such as blogs, podcasts, social media, and online publications [2]. For more information on altmetrics see Chap. 6. By incorporating altmetrics, many publishers are recognizing the importance of online social media role in scholarly publication and therefore playing a major role in the tenure and promotion process [3].

Incorporating altmetrics into a scholars' overall impact metrics is growing in popularity and acceptance. By measuring activities such as social bookmarking, blog mentions, additions to reference managers, etc., of scholarly articles, a more complete picture of an academics' research and impact can be formed. The greatest challenges and limitations for promotion and tenure committees entail assessing the quality and the impact of scholarly work using social media. An important aspect of digital scholarship is the growing effort to establish digital and social media as credible, professional, and legitimate means of scholarship and communication.

The increasing acceptance from academic institutions, publishers, and colleagues demonstrates the growing importance of online social media. Promotion and tenure guidelines will need to be updated which will no doubt encourage more scholars to use these tools in the future. This will also allow institutions to develop high quality academic standards.

Personal Branding or Self-Promotion vs. Organizational Promotion

Your motivations should dictate how, when and where you become involved with digital platforms. Decide how you want to be portrayed and be consistent across the platforms you choose. Deciding why you want to be on social media or academic networking sites can help you design and curate your digital identity.

To have a public face and digital identity that belongs to both an individual and an institution requires an understanding of how to manage online behaviors and experiences. This is still relatively new, despite the availability of many social media platforms for the last two decades. The personal perspective of using social media professionally may vary depending on the individual (Fig. 10.1).

Academics must learn to align their personal interests with their professional responsibilities and goals on any digital platform. Many institutions place an increasingly greater value on online professional representation, and the need to protect themselves from negative publicity [4]. It is suggested that you familiarize yourself with your organization social media policies before establishing a digital identity on any platform.

Your motivations should dictate how and where you become involved with social media. Decide how you want to be portrayed and be consistent across the platforms you choose. The growth of participation in social media and ASNS usage for

Why Do You Want to Increase Your Online Presence?
- To get a job?
- To raise the visibility of your book or research?
- To find out about interesting trends in your field?
- Foster conversation with your students?
- Identify who is your audience?
- What do you hope to learn from and contribute to other communities?
- Are you hoping to identify other collaborators?

Fig. 10.1 Why increase your online presence [1]

self-branding and promotion, rather than for the profile of the university or organization, can be confusing for those outside looking in. Academics should always disclose a conflict of interest.

Maintain the Integrity of the ORCID Registry

Many research publications request or require that authors register for an ORCID during the manuscript submission process and before publication. This is done so each author can secure a unique persistent identifier as they engage in research and scholarship. This reflects the mission of ORCID to "connect research and researchers" [5].

Recently the accuracy or transparency of the ORCID registry has been called into question [6]. There have been issues with misinformation and the quality of some records. ORCID can be used by fraudulent authors, or by others creating fake researcher accounts for unethical purposes. The existence of ghost ORCID accounts in which information is missing or unreliable reduces the ability of verifying if the researcher is truly who they say they are [5]. These faulty entries may call into question the quality of the ORCID infrastructure and may fuel the rise of detractors and skepticism about the service [6].

As outlined in Chapter 4, the ability to verify authorship and transparency is vital to the academic community. Managing and curating your personal ORCID record is vital to maintaining the integrity of the ORCID registry.

Harassment

Will increased transparency by using digital profiles on ASNS and social media reduce harassment of women, minorities, LGBTQIA+ and other groups? Will it cut down on harassment of researchers that work in the fields of sexuality, climate research and politics?

The popularity of X, or Twitter, and other social media platforms can pose a challenge for professors and administrators. Educators often find it useful to disseminate their work, but it can reflect on the school if their research or opinions are controversial. Sometimes academics can create controversy with potentially offensive tweets [7]. While some academics have managed to leverage their use of social media into greater public knowledge of their research, others worry about using social media, fearing that any potentially offensive speech or any other slip-up may not only reflect poorly on them, but on their work [7].

Many tenured professors are hesitant to speak out forcefully on social media platforms, but the danger is even greater for adjunct professors, as well as part-time and non-tenure track full time professors. They are not afforded the protections that are provided to tenured professors.

Others may argue that if universities attempt to limit the freedom of speech and ideas online, it could harm the integrity of the learning environment. It is a delicate balancing act for administrators, who need to implement or to develop policies and guidelines that protect the institutions reputation along with the opinions of the faculty they employee [7].

Some researchers and academics have expressed concern for the institutional lack of control or responsibility for external social media tools and the potential issues of cyberbullying, unprofessional behavior, and lack of privacy. Academics and researchers using any social platforms need to be professional and respectful.

Being transparent with your digital profile will cut down on harassment and improve online safety. By making your digital profile more transparent you are discouraging a negative culture on that platform. You are promoting a more tolerant and respectful online environment. Adopting transparent practices and stricter university guidelines should reduce internal and external harassment and discrimination.

Future Academics

Will the next generation of researchers and academics know how to separate private from public identities in social platforms? An exceedingly important aspect of academic development and promotion is your reputation. Reputation can greatly be impacted by social and digital media. It is very important to carefully monitor your online presence.

In the past, career centers offered workshops on resume development and cover letter advice. Today's students are establishing a digital footprint earlier in their careers, so it is important to curate their digital presence early on.

It is important to establish instruction, in a student's academic career, for them to understand the importance of separating personal and professional digital identities. One way this can be conducted is through instruction by librarians, instructional designers, and professors in all fields. For example, students should be instructed on how best to design a professional LinkedIn profile. This should include instruction on how to locate and use the privacy settings on each platform. It can include instructions on how to evaluate their current online presence with suggestions on how to assess and clean it up. Discussions can follow that would elaborate on specific parameters that would educate students on what to keep private on their digital profile.

Upcoming researchers and academics should be made aware of regulatory guidelines that need to be followed in their professional careers. Students must be aware that there could be consequences of establishing their presence on digital platforms. Boundaries should be understood between what is shared publicly and what should remain private [8].

Guidelines

Will more professional organizations issue guidelines or recommendations on using social media and maintaining a professional presence in the digital world? In 2021, the American Medical Association (AMA) issued guidelines in its code of medical ethics titled, Professionalism in the Use of Social Media [9]. This guideline recognizes the importance a professional presence online for physicians, residents and students by introducing the issues that they should be aware of such as: privacy, confidentiality, appropriate boundaries of the patient/physician relationship, and the consequences that can negatively affect their reputations among patients and colleagues [8].

Academics and researchers who use digital platforms for their scholarship and dissemination of their work, need to uphold the policies of their institutions. Your digital presence should also meet the standards of any professional organization you have an active membership with. Professional ethics should be practiced while disseminating ideas, interactions, opinions, or research while online.

Conclusion

There are some current trends on the use of academic networking or social media platforms that ultimately revolve around two recurring themes: first, potential benefits to the academic community; and second, reservations expressed by scholars.

Your research presence in today's digital environment is no longer seen as supplemental or optional. Developing and maintaining a digital presence is seen as an essential component and extension of your professional work and reputation.

Having a digital profile to clearly identify you as an author and your affiliated research is vital and necessary to the integrity of scholarship. The decision to jump into the world of digital and social media platforms is one that should be well planned. There are benefits and risks when exploring and establishing a digital identity.

This book explored issues that should be considered before establishing or maintaining a digital identity (Fig. 10.2). Librarians can educate academics on their digital profiles by sharing their expertise in areas such as author rights, self-archiving, and alternative metrics. By increasing awareness of these issues, librarians will be educating and supporting their colleagues to correctly use these digital platforms.

A strong online identity is important for researchers and scholars in the digital age. A digital identity represents researchers' online presence and reputation in the research community. It makes their scholarship visible and helps them gain more recognition as they publicize and share their work. To assist in that, ORCiD, a persistent digital identifier, is increasingly being used and promoted to make research more visible, discoverable, accessible, and recognizable.

Tips…

Familiarize yourself with your institution or professional organizations "best practice recommendations".

Attend workshops at your instition that focus on developing and maintaing a digital presence. Academics and students need to be taught the best ways digital identies are formed and maintained

Be aware of social media policies and ask about them if they aren't mentioned during new student or faculty orientation.

Understand the tensions between professional and personal information that may reflect poorly on your or your organization.

Continue to educate yourself and new colleagues about the impact and permenance of the digital footprint.[8]

Fig. 10.2 Tips on digital profiles [8]

Understanding the concepts of author and alternative metrics and their impact is important in establishing your research identity and your professional achievements. Understanding how these metrics represent your digital identity can be used to measure or improve your academic output. Having these metrics available allows scholars to achieve promotion, tenure, and funding opportunities.

Developing a solid digital foundation, such as a professional website, to highlight your career achievements is another step in establishing your digital presence. A website can make you more recognizable and increase your networking reach. Social media also plays an important role in establishing one's digital identity. There are a variety of platforms to use that will allow you to engage with fellow colleagues and disseminate your research. How you use social media will determine your reputation in your field. Guidelines and best practices will help you establish a strong footing for your digital profile.

Academics who do establish a digital profile on ASNS or social media platforms can become overwhelmed by the demands, leading them to either avoid updating their profiles or letting them sit dormant. Although many networking sites claim that they have a profound impact on scholarly research and career goals, some scholars report experiencing information overload and others doubt the need for any digital platforms.

The real concern is a lack of know-how relative to using specific platforms in order to achieve positive outcomes and develop a professional reputation. Since academic social networks are continuously evolving, it is necessary for researchers to stay current on issues such as platform updates and changes in use, particularly among their peers [10]. Establishing a clear and concise digital profile can only benefit you and your career.

Navigating the field in this digital environment will be bumpy, filled with holes and no road maps. As technology grows so will social media and academic social networking sites. There will be more platforms available to learn and to use. For many in academics there will be a period of learning and adjustment as we become more familiar with the new technology. We remain optimistic about the future of digital academic platforms. A greater understanding will emerge as scholars and researchers continue to share and study the successes and challenges of utilizing digital social networking.

References

1. O'Regan A, Smithson WH, Spain E. Social media and professional identity: pitfalls and potential. Med Teach. 2018;40(2):112–6. https://doi.org/10.1080/0142159X.2017.1396308.
2. Johng SY, Mishori R, Korostyshevskiy VR. Social media, digital scholarship, and academic promotion in US Medical Schools. Fam Med. 2021;53(3):215–9. https://doi.org/10.22454/FamMed.2021.146684.
3. Cabrera D, Vartabedian BS, Spinner RJ, Jordan BL, Aase LA, Timimi FK. More than likes and tweets: creating social media portfolios for academic promotion and tenure. J Grad Med Educ. 2017;9(4):421–5. https://doi.org/10.4300/jgme-d-17-00171.1.
4. Pruvis AJ, Rogers HM, Beckingham S. Experiences and perspectives of social media in learning and teaching in higher education. Int J Educ Res Open. 2020;1:100018. https://doi.org/10.1016/j.ijedro.2020.100018.
5. Teixeira da Silva JA. Non-compliance with ethical rules caused by misuse of ORCID accounts: implications for medical publications in the COVID-19 era. Ethics Med Public Health. 2021;18:100692. https://doi.org/10.1016/j.jemep.2021.100692.
6. Baglioni M, Manghi P, Mannocci A, Bardi A. We can make a better use of ORCID: five observed misapplications. Data Sci J. 2021;20:38. https://doi.org/10.5334/dsj-2021-038.
7. Donachie P. Social media use remains thorny issue for academics and colleges. 2017. https://www.highereddive.com/news/social-media-use-remains-thorny-issue-for-academics-and-colleges/442619/. Accessed 20 Nov 2022.
8. Marshal M, Niranjan V, Spain E, MacDonagh J, O'Doherty J, O'Connor R, et al. 'Doctors can't be doctors all of the time': a qualitative study of how general practitioners and medical students negotiate public-professional and private-personal realms using social media. BMJ Open. 2021;11(10):e047991. https://doi.org/10.1136/bmjopen-2020-047991.
9. American Medical Association. Professionalism in the use of social media. Chicago: AMA; 2021.
10. Williams AE, Woodacre MA. The possibilities and perils of academic social networking sites. Online Inf Rev. 2016;40(2):282–94. https://doi.org/10.1108/OIR-10-2015-0327.

Correction to: Tools for Managing Your Digital Research Identity

Layal Hneiny

Correction to: Chapter 5 in: M. R. Dreker, K. J. Downey (eds.), *Building Your Academic Research Digital Identity. A Step-Wise Guide to Cultivating Your Academic Research Career Online*, https://doi.org/10.1007/978-3-031-50317-7_5

Owing to an unfortunate oversight, the book was inadvertently published with incorrect figures in Chapter 5.

The corrections are listed below.

1. Figures 5.3, 5.7, and 5.8 had been incorrectly published, which are now replaced with correct figures.

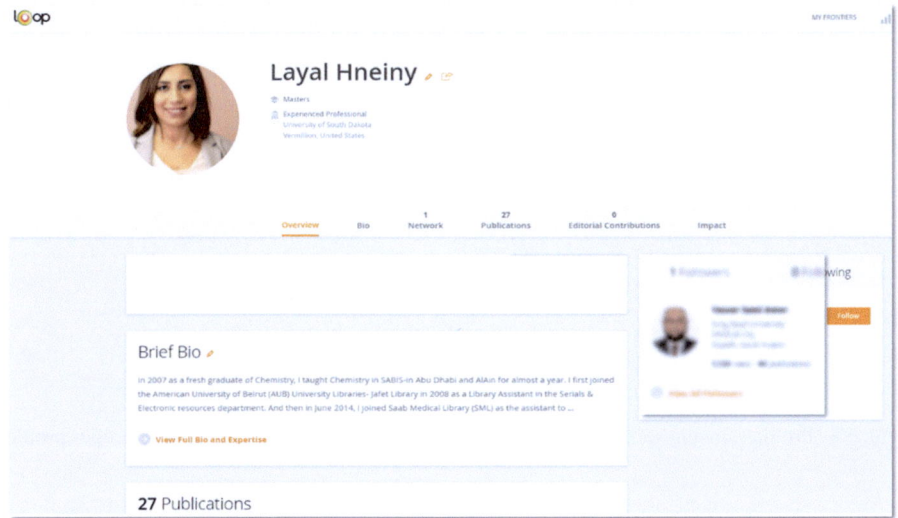

Fig. 5.3 A glimpse into the overview in Loop's platform

The updated version of this chapter can be found at https://doi.org/10.1007/978-3-031-50317-7_5

© The Author(s), under exclusive license to Springer Nature Switzerland AG 2024
M. R. Dreker, K. J. Downey (eds.), *Building Your Academic Research Digital Identity*, https://doi.org/10.1007/978-3-031-50317-7_11

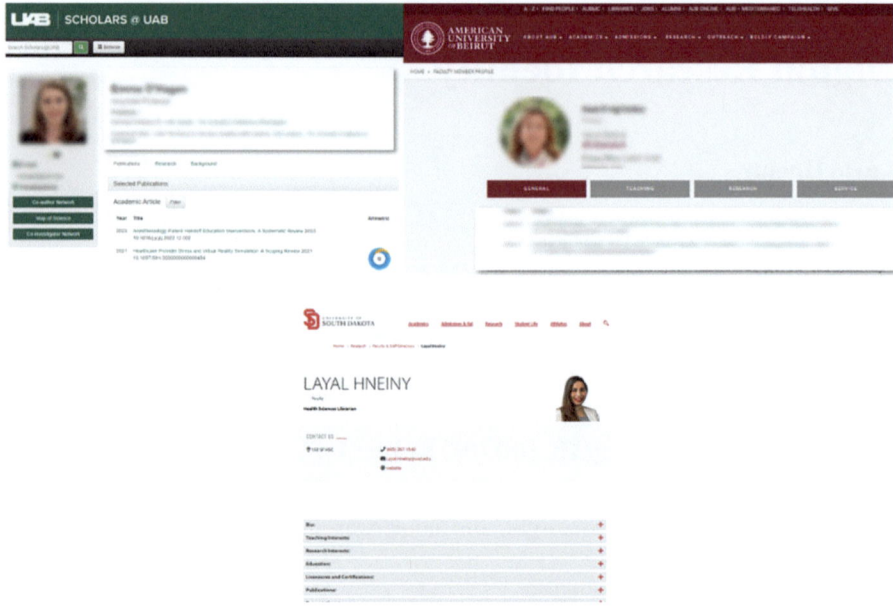

Fig. 5.7 Different profiles of different faculty from different universities

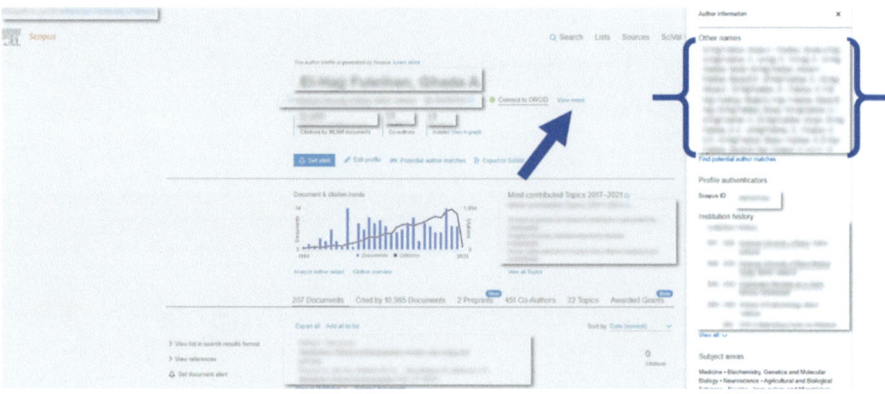

Fig. 5.8 Profile showing variations of names for the same researcher in her unique Scopus profile

Index

A
Academic career, 146
Academic librarians, 24
Academic Social Networks Sites (ASNS), 2, 9
Altmetric attention score, 65
Altmetric badge, 65
Altmetrics, 6, 13, 26, 65
    analysis, 59
    course limitations, 80
    databases, e-journal platforms, 80
    definition, 78
    tools, 65
American Medical Association (AMA) guidelines, 147
Author ID, 62
Author Impact Factor (AIF), 70
Author metrics, 69
    Author Impact Factor (AIF), 74
    bibliographic databases, 75
    e-index, 73
    g-index, 73
    Google Scholar, 77
    H-index, 71
    i10-index, 74
    quantification of research, 70
    Scopus, 76
    traditional metrics, 78
    Web of Science (WoS), 75
Author profiles, 85

B
Banner images, 104
Berlin declaration, 32
Bibliometrics, 13

C
Colleague online harassment, 135
Conference platforms, 94
Curation, 121–122
Cyberbullying, 132–133

D
Data repository, 94
Digital identity, 1, 2, 4, 9, 35, 93
    academic career, 91–92
    academic identity, 17
    ASNS, 9
    authorship, 10
    digital profile, 17
    gain visibility, 18
    high-ranking sites, 16
    names, 11
    ORCID, 15, 18, 20
    privacy settings, 19
    publish/perish, 10
    researchers, 36
    research funding agencies, 15
    social media platforms, 16
    social platforms, 19
    STEM fields, 11
    unique identifier, 14
Digital platform(s), 3, 97
Digital profile, 11, 12
Digital transformation, 5
DMPTool, 44
Doximity profile, 56

F
Facebook
  feed, 119
  functions, 119
  groups, 120
  overview, 118
  posts, 120
  profile, 119
Findable, accessible, interoperable, reusable (FAIR), 92
Florida State University (FSU) School, 88

G
Google Scholar (GS) profiles, 63

H
Handle harassment, 135
Harassment, 145–146
Hashtags, 122
H-index, 59
  classical bibliometric indicator, 72
  scientific community, 71

I
Identity, 1
Infrastructure, 142
Instagram
  biography, 117
  function, 115
  image filters, 116
  links, 117
  overview, 115
  posts, 117–118
  profile, 116
  reels, 116
  stories, 116
  videos, 116, 118
Institutional repositories, 52
Interprofessional Health Science (IHS) library, 29
Inter-University Consortium for Political and Social Research (ICPSR), 29

L
Librarians, 5, 24
Libraries, 23
LinkedIn, 55, 104
  additional group, 107
  build connections, 108
  comments, 108
  featured section, 107
  functions, 104–105
  groups, 109
  interest groups, 106
  multimedia capabilities, 105
  name pronunciation, 108
  posts, 106, 109
  premium subscription, 106
  profile tips, 106
  profile views, 12, 105
Loop, 54

N
National Science Foundation (NSF), 85

O
Online harassment, 133–134
Online hate, 134
Open access (OA) publishing, 31, 32, 86
Open Researcher and Contributor ID (ORCID), 5, 29, 36, 37
  benefits, 38, 39
  bioksketch format pages, 43
  definition, 37
  delegation, 45
  digital identifier, 37
  DMPTool, 43
  NSPM-33 guidance, 41
  ORCID iD, 37
  profile, 91
  record, 45
  registry, 40, 145
  stakeholders' requirements, 40–42
Open science
  academic career, 88
  article processing charges (APC), 88
  definition, 87
  equitable business models, 88
  open access, 87
  personal website, 89
Organization tools, 94

P
Personal Academic Website, 90–91, 97
Plagiarism, 130
PlumX gathers, 80
PlumX metrics, 31
Privacy, 142
Professional digital presence, 18–19

Professional organizations, 96
Profile upkeep, 121–122
Promotion, 142–144
Publication metrics, 69
Public writing, 3
PubMed profile, 53

R
ResearcherID number, 62
ResearchGate(RG), 57, 109
    disciplines, 111
    functions, 110
    messages, 111
    profile, 111
    question and answer posts, 110, 111
    research, 112
    score, 110
    skills and expertise, 112
    upload articles, 110
Research information management systems (RIMS), 36

S
Scholarly communication, 27
Scholarly Publishing and Academic Resources Coalition (SPARC), 87
Science Experts Network Curriculum Vitae (SciENcv), 42
Science, technology, engineering, and mathematics (STEM) fields, 11
Scopus, 60, 76
    author profile, 76
    course limitations, 76
Scouting content, 122
Secure socket layer (SSL), 88
Self-promotion *vs.* organizational promotion, 144–145
Seton Hall University, (SHU) librarians, 28, 30
SHU eRepository, 30
Social and ethical issues, 141
Social media, 4, 6, 9, 12, 101
    accounts, 137
    digital profile, 102–103

    email account, 103
    profile picture, 103
Social media platform(s), 3, 102, 121, 127
    active user, 122
    addictive properties, 123
    colleagues, 123
    digital profile, 128
    enough, 124
    profile pictures, 128–129
    security risks, 129
    spell check feature, 123
Software robots, 124

T
Tenure, 142–144
Trolling, 136
Twitter, 64, 112
    biography, 115
    default handles, 115
    disclaimers, 20
    followers, 113
    function, 112–113
    poll feature, 114
    protected tweets, 113
    threads, 114
    tweets, 113
    verified accounts, 114
    video tweets, 114
    website, 115

U
University of Houston (UH) Libraries, 25
University of Minnesota (UMN) Libraries, 26–28
University Webpages, 58–59

W
Web of Science (WoS), 75
Wikipedia, 64

MIX
Papier aus verantwortungsvollen Quellen
Paper from responsible sources
FSC® C105338

If you have any concerns about our products,
you can contact us on
ProductSafety@springernature.com

In case Publisher is established outside the EU,
the EU authorized representative is:
**Springer Nature Customer Service Center GmbH
Europaplatz 3, 69115 Heidelberg, Germany**

Printed by Libri Plureos GmbH
in Hamburg, Germany